W9-DHR-722

Lifetime Fitness

Fourth Edition

H. Larry Brown

North Carolina State University

Contributing Authors:

Louis Almekinders   Charles Raynor
Sally Almekinders   Tom Roberts
Jim DeWitt   Timothy Winslow
Bob Gwyn   George Youtt

ALLYN AND BACON
BOSTON LONDON TORONTO SYDNEY TOKYO SINGAPORE

Copyright © 1996, 1992, 1989, 1986
by Allyn and Bacon
A Viacom Company
Needham Heights, Massachusetts 02194

Internet: www.abacon.com
America Online: keyword: College Online

All rights reserved. No part of the material
protected by this copyright notice may be
reproduced or utilized in any form or by any
means, electronic or mechanical, including
photocopying, recording, or by any information
storage and retrieval system, without the written
permission of the copyright owner.

ISBN 0-13-776618-1

Printed in the United States of America

10 9 8 7 6 5 4 3 2   01 00 99 98 97

Contents

Chapter 6   Nutrition and Health   81

Chapter 7   Body Composition and Weight Control   97

Chapter 8   Stress Management   113

Appendix A Exercise-Related Injuries   121

Appendix B: Fitness Forms   125

Index   143

Preface

Good health and fitness are the cornerstones of a productive, healthy, and happy life. Like the three previous editions of this text, this new fourth edition of *Lifetime Fitness* will help students understand the benefits of exercise and proper nutrition. The information in this book offers readers a concise but thorough overview of the many factors contributing to the development and maintenance of a healthy body.

Lifetime Fitness will help students evaluate their levels of fitness, including cardiorespiratory fitness, which plays an essential role in overall good health. Students can design personalized exercise programs to achieve their specific goals. The text includes step-by-step instructions for many exercises and accompanying photographs. In addition, the book identifies problems and injuries that participants may encounter during training and suggests safety measures to avoid them.

An expanded and updated nutrition chapter provides detailed information about nutrients and their functions, as well as current consumption guidelines for fat, protein, and carbohydrates. A separate chapter on body composition and weight control allows students to determine lean and fat body-weight percentages; it also includes a formula for calculating desired body weight.

The final chapter of the book discusses stress—the causes, the symptoms, the results, and what can be done to reduce the stresses of everyday life. The chapter includes a three-part "stress test" developed by the U.S. Department of Health and Human Services. Review questions follow each chapter.

Appendices for the book again include a preexercise medical and fitness information form, fitness evaluation records, and a cardiorespiratory start sheet as well as a new appendix on exercise-related injuries. The forms provided help instructors evaluate student participants accurately and efficiently. As before, the book also includes charts to help students track cardiorespiratory progress and improvements in muscular strength and endurance.

The health and fitness programs students choose today will have a major impact on their future lifestyles. Using the information in *Lifetime Fitness*, students can design programs that will be both fun and productive.

Acknowledgments

I wish to thank the following authors for their help in making *Lifetime Fitness* the concise, up-to-date book it is: Louis Almekinders, Sally Almekinders, Jim DeWitt, Bob Gwyn, Charles Raynor, Tom Roberts, Timothy Winslow, and George Youtt.

I would especially like to thank Dr. Louis Almekinders, who is an orthopedic surgeon, for writing Appendix A, Exercise-Related Injuries. His expertise in this area will be extremely beneficial for our readers.

I would also like to thank the reviewers of this and previous editions, who offered constructive, helpful suggestions; they include Charles Linn of Evangel College, Tim Gleeson of Southwestern Michigan College, Anita Erdman of Harrisburg Area Community College, Carolyn M. Mauck of Del Mar College, and Marvene Wallace of Texas Southmost College. Finally, thanks to all of you who use the book and have provided positive feedback and suggestions for its continued improvement.

1

Introduction

Why follow a program of lifetime fitness? The best reason for most people is that it promotes a happier, more fulfilling, and more productive life. When a brilliant but obese, stress-laden, heavy-smoking, and physically inactive individual is unable to work or dies from a heart attack during middle age, a human resource is lost. While it is difficult to prove that being fit will lengthen your lifespan, we are certain that fitness does improve the quality of life. Evidence overwhelmingly indicates that our learning potential, within our given level of intelligence, increases in accordance with our level of physical fitness. A gradual reduction of functional capacity for thought, work, and recreation will occur if you allow yourself to succumb to the ease and comfort of today's electronic, push-button world. However, an active lifestyle will enable you to enjoy the comforts of modern technology without losing functional capacity.

Keeping fit and practicing good health habits are your responsibilities. Your future health and well-being depend largely upon the lifestyle you are now developing. This book will help you understand the principles of fitness and apply these concepts to your own plan for lifetime fitness.

PHYSICAL FITNESS

Physical fitness is often defined as the ability to perform daily physical tasks energetically and still have energy reserves to perform recreational activities and respond to emergencies requiring strength and stamina. Fitness is not merely being well or not being sick. All people exhibit some level of physical fitness; this state is minimal in the severely ill and much greater in the highly conditioned individual.

Very few individuals extend the effort to reach their maximum potential, although many are able to improve their fitness level. A common fallacy is to equate athletic ability—the ability to perform specific sport skills—with physical fitness. It is true that the majority of highly trained athletes are physically fit, but this does not imply that you must possess athletic ability in order to achieve a high level of fitness. Many individuals who have attained high fitness levels through regular participation in well-planned fitness programs are not, and never have been, skilled athletes. There are also numerous examples of individuals who have mastered certain athletic skills and yet are not physically fit. This book will be beneficial in helping you set realistic goals for yourself. As you set your goals, avoid comparing yourself and your accomplishments to other people and their accomplishments. Achieve *your* goals, not someone else's.

COMPONENTS OF FITNESS

The five components of fitness are **flexibility, cardiorespiratory capacity, muscular strength, muscular endurance,** and **body composition.**

Flexibility.   Flexibility is the functional capacity of a joint to move through a normal range of motion. Flexibility is highly specific and depends largely upon the muscles and connective tissue *surrounding* the joint, although arthritis and other bone diseases certainly do affect the joint itself. Good flexibility is characterized by freedom of movement and contributes to ease and economy of muscular effort.

Cardiorespiratory Capacity.   Cardiorespiratory (CR) capacity is the functional capacity of the heart, lungs, and blood vessels to take in and deliver oxygen to the aerobic working muscles. Generally, exercisers develop CR fitness through sustained endurance activities such as running, swimming, cycling, rowing, cross-country skiing, and others that require the use of large-muscle groups in a rhythmic fashion for an extended period of time, including at least 15 minutes (preferably 30) of vigorous activity.

Muscular Strength.   Muscular strength is the maximum amount of force a muscle or group of muscles can exert during one contraction. Muscular strength, in its purest form, is utilized in activities requiring the exertion of maximum force in a *single, all-out effort.* Lifting a barbell one time with as much weight on it as you can lift is an example. Most activities, however, require more than a single maximum effort and are a combination of muscular strength and endurance.

Muscular Endurance.   Muscular endurance is the ability of a muscle or group of muscles to exert force for an extended period of time. Strength and muscular endurance are directly related but are at opposite ends of the strength–endurance training continuum. The more times you repeat a muscular movement, the closer you are to the endurance end of the continuum.

Body Composition.   Body composition refers to the amount of body fat and lean body mass you have. Many Americans have too much body fat (are overfat) due to their sedentary lifestyles and their consumption of too much fat in their diets. Body fat for men should not comprise more than 15 to 18 percent of the total body weight, and body fat for women should comprise no more than 25 to 28 percent of the total body weight.

A good fitness program includes activities that will develop all fitness components. Adequate rest and a balanced diet are also important in order to obtain desired results. Practically anyone can become fit; the only requirements are time and dedication.

ENTRANCE EVALUATION

You should evaluate your present condition prior to participating in a regular fitness program. First identify any medical problems you may have. If you do have any medical problems or are over the age of 35, you should receive a medical examination before beginning a fitness program. If you have no medical restrictions, evaluate yourself on a few performance tests to establish your level in each of the five components of fitness.

Flexibility. Many tests measure flexibility. One of the most commonly used is the **sit-and-reach test,** which measures the flexibility of the hip extensors and lower back. Lack of flexibility in these areas, combined with poor strength in the abdominal and hip-flexor muscles can lead to chronic back pain. The procedures for administering the test are found in Chapter 3 and norms for college students are listed in Table 3.1.

CR Capacity. The most accurate method to determine the cardiorespiratory fitness of an individual is to measure oxygen consumption using a graded-exercise stress test. However, this method is both time-consuming and costly. Therefore, the **step test** and the 1.5-mile run are often used when testing large groups of healthy individuals.

The step test consists of stepping up and down on a bench, the height of which is 14 inches for women and 18 inches for men, at a rate of 120 steps per minute for three minutes (time 0:00 to 3:00). The movement of each foot, up or down, counts as one step. At the end of three minutes, the participant sits down and locates the radial pulse (on the wrist, near the base of the thumb) within ten seconds (time 3:01 to 3:10). It is beneficial to have another counter find the carotid pulse while you are finding your radial pulse. To locate the carotid pulse, place two fingers on your Adam's apple and then slide them into the groove alongside the Adam's apple. Do *not* use your thumb to locate either the radial or carotid pulse. It is extremely important that the individual taking the carotid pulse does not press down firmly, as this may decrease the blood supply to the brain. The pulse count is then taken for 15 seconds (time 3:11 to 3:25) and recorded. You then take your pulse rate two more times (from time 4:11 to 4:25 and from 5:11 to 5:25). Normally, the fitter you are, the lower each score will be. Also, if you exercise regularly, the change between the first and second counts will be greater than the change between the second and third counts. Norms for the step test are given in Tables 1.1 and 1.2.

The time it takes to run 1.5 miles is also often used to measure cardiorespiratory fitness. We suggest using the step test rather than the 1.5-mile run as an entrance evaluation method if you are not moderately conditioned before entering a fitness program. Many fitness programs do not utilize the 1.5-mile run as an entrance test because of the difficulty untrained individuals have in judging pace. Table 4.2 in Chapter 4 lists the norms for the 1.5-mile run.

Muscular Strength. As mentioned earlier, muscular strength is the maximum amount of force that you can exert during one contraction. A valid test of muscular strength is the bench press. To test yourself, read the instructions in Chapter 5 and look at Figures 5.1 and 5.2. Find the weight that you are sure you can press more than one time. Use spotters and press the weight as many times as possible. Do not hold your breath while lifting. After determining how many times you can lift a particular weight, you need to compute the maximum weight you could have lifted one time. To compute the maximum weight, use the Brown formula:

Maximum Weight = [(Repetitions × .0328 + .9849) × Resistance]

For example, if you lifted a weight of 150 pounds six times, you would compute your maximum weight:

[(6 × .0328 + .9849) × 150] = 177 pounds

Tables 1.1 and 1.2 include norms for the bench press. To determine how you compare against other students, compare the maximum weight you can lift to your body weight. For instance, in the example above your maximum weight was 177 pounds. If you weigh 140 pounds, the ratio of your maximum weight compared to your body weight will be 177:140, which gives you a ratio of 1.26. According to Table 1.1, this would place you within the 80–90 percentile. Many fitness programs will use test items that measure a combination of muscular strength and endurance as a strength assessment in order to avoid injuries that may occur when testing untrained individuals in a single, all-out effort.

Muscular Endurance.   In addition to being a test for muscular strength, the bench press may be used to test muscular endurance as long as the resistance (amount of weight being lifted) is light. If you are a young man you can use 75 percent of your body weight and 33 percent of your body weight if you are a young woman. After determining how much weight you should use, perform the exercise as many times as possible. Be sure to use good form and have spotters. Tables 1.1 and 1.2 list the norms for college-age students.

Body Composition.   You should record your body weight and fat percentage before beginning your training program. The procedure for measuring your fat percentage is discussed in Chapter 7. Table 7.1 gives classifications of body composition according to fat percentage, while Tables 7.2 and 7.3 help you determine your fat percentage.

TEST RESULTS AND THEIR MEANINGS

The norms for the preceding tests for college students are listed in Tables 1.1 and 1.2. This information allows you to compare your test results to those of approximately 36,000 men and 9,000 women tested at North Carolina State University.

These results will give you a starting point for maintaining a progression record. You should not be concerned about your current percentile. However, it is important to keep track of your performance level as you progress. Be concerned with your goals, not your past record. The Preexercise Medical and Fitness Information form in Appendix B can be used to record some of your entrance evaluation scores.

Table 1.1   **Entrance evaluation norms for men.**

PERCENTILE	STRENGTH BENCH*	ENDURANCE BENCH**	STEP EoT	STEP +1	STEP +2
99	1.60	35	15	12	12
90	1.32	23	30	22	19
80	1.20	18	33	24	21
70	1.12	15	34	26	22.5
60	1.05	13	35	27.5	24
50	.99	10	36.5	29	25
40	.93	7	37.5	30	27
30	.87	5	38.5	32	27.5
20	.81	3	40	34	28.5
10	.74	<1	41.5	41	30.5

*The value is the ratio of the maximum weight one can lift to his body weight.
**The value is the number of repetitions performed with 75 percent of body weight.

Table 1.2 Entrance evaluation norms for women.

PERCENTILE	STRENGTH BENCH*	ENDURANCE BENCH**	STEP EoT	STEP +1	STEP +2
99	.735	37	18	13	12.5
90	.520	18	33	22.5	19.5
80	.488	15	35	26	22
70	.462	12	36	27.5	24
60	.438	10	37	29	25.5
50	.419	8	38	30	26.5
40	.400	7	39	31	27.5
30	.380	5	40	32.5	29
20	.354	2	41	33.5	29.5
10	.322	<1	42.5	35	31

*The value is the ratio of the maximum weight one can lift to her body weight.
**The value is the number of repetitions performed with 33 percent of body weight.

Note: For Tables 1.1 and 1.2,
   EoT refers to pulse count at end of test.
   +1 refers to pulse count one minute after completion of test.
   +2 refers to pulse count two minutes after completion of test.

SUPPLEMENTARY READINGS

Allsen, P. E., J. M. Harrison, and B. Vance. *Fitness for Life: An Individualized Approach.* 5th ed. Madison, WI: Brown & Benchmark, 1993.

Harris, D. V., and J. A. Peterson. *Personal Fitness Guide.* Englewood, CO: Morton Publishing Company, 1988.

Hoeger, W. W. K. *Lifetime Physical Fitness.* 3d ed. Englewood, CO: Morton Publishing Company, 1992.

Marley, W. P. *Health & Physical Fitness.* Dubuque, IA: Wm. C. Brown, 1988.

Mazzeo, K. *A Commitment to Fitness.* Englewood, CO: Morton Publishing Company, 1985.

CHAPTER 1 REVIEW QUESTIONS

1. List three benefits of being physically fit.

    a.

    b.

    c.

2. Define physical fitness.

3. List and define the five components of fitness. Also, for each component of fitness, list a test that you can use to measure your present fitness level for that component.

    a.

    b.

    c.

    d.

    e.

4. What precautions should you take before starting a fitness program?

2

Safety and Training Considerations

This chapter will identify training principles and guidelines that you should consider before participating in a training program. Careful attention to these principles and guidelines not only will help to ensure your safety but also will maximize your results from the training program.

As mentioned in Chapter 1, if you are over the age of 35 or have any medical problems, you should receive clearance form a physician before participating in an exercise program. It is also important to consider your physical limitations when deciding on the type of activities your program will include. For example, if you are overweight, start with a walking or swimming program before participating in a jogging program. Your choice of activity is referred to as the **mode** of exercise. If you experience breathing difficulty, chest pain, persistent pain, dizziness, or nausea at any time during your exercise program, terminate the exercise and consult a physician.

TRAINING PRINCIPLES AND GUIDELINES

In order to achieve desired results from your training program, you should understand the training principles and guidelines discussed in this chapter. The acronym **SPORT FIT** will help you to remember these training principles and guidelines. **SPORT** refers to the training principles of Specificity, Progression, Overload, Reversibility, and Training Individuality. **FIT** refers to the training guidelines of Frequency, Intensity, and Time.

Specificity.   Training is specific to the cells, and to the structural and functional elements within the cells, that are overloaded. Transfer of training occurs only to the extent that you recruit the same motor units and use them in a similar manner. A motor unit consists of a motor neuron with all the muscle cells it innervates. When attempting to increase your muscular strength and endurance for a given activity, it is best to perform the movement required in the activity against resistance. If the nature of the activity does not permit this, then the major muscle groups involved in the activity should be trained using progressive-resistance exercises as similar as possible to the movement of the activity. The development of muscular strength and endurance depends upon the type, frequency, intensity, and amount of exercise performed.

Progression.   As physiological adaptations from training take place in the body, you will experience a sensation of reduced effort for a given performance. This is due to the adaptations enhancing your ability to remove metabolic by-products and replace energy. In order to continue overloading your system for steady improvement, increase your training intensity. This will be a continual process in your training program.

Overload.   In order for a muscle cell to increase in size (hypertrophy) and strength, you must increase the cell's workload beyond what it normally experiences. Furthermore, once a muscle adapts to a higher workload, further strength gains require additional increases in workload. This overload principle is the underlying concept of progressive-resistance training.

Reversibility.   Even though you may have a high level of fitness, you must continue a regular program of training in order to avoid deconditioning. A significant reduction of working capacity begins to occur within two weeks after cessation of training. The saying "Use it or lose it" certainly applies to physical fitness. The effects of training are transient and depend on continued training. Cessation of training results in a gradual decline of performance capacity and a decrease in size (atrophy) of the adapted muscle cells.

Training Individuality.   Although research studies attempt to describe the typical person, individuals respond differently to precise physiological responses, and adaptations will vary slightly from individual to individual. Tailor your program to meet your needs, and be sure to listen to your body when training.

Frequency, Intensity, Time (FIT).   Your body needs to receive a training stimulus every 36 to 48 hours at a level that meets the overload requirements for a sufficient amount of time in order for your fitness level to improve or remain high. In strength training, a training stimulus every other day is preferable. In cardiorespiratory activities, training is generally recommended three to five days a week for weight-bearing activities such as jogging or running, and five to seven days a week for non-weight-bearing activities such as cycling or swimming. Training more than five days a week in weight-bearing activities often results in overuse injuries. However, it is possible to train seven days a week without overuse injuries if you use a variety of activities for cardiorespiratory training. For example, you could swim and jog on alternating days and probably train seven days a week without injuries from overuse.

The intensity of the exercise should be sufficient to overload the body. For cardiorespiratory training, the intensity should be between 60 to 90 percent of your maximum heart rate reserve (see Chapter 4). The intensity should be approximately 60 to 80 percent of your maximum effort for muscular strength and endurance training (see Chapter 5). However, if you are just starting the training program, *always* start at a low intensity and stay with a low intensity during the first few weeks of training. For optimal results, your workout schedule should alternate difficult and easy days, instead of each workout day being progressively harder. Your training schedule should resemble a sawtooth instead of a linear graph in regard to intensity and time.

The time of the workout session should be 20 to 60 minutes of continuous training for the cardiorespiratory activity and enough time to exercise the major muscle groups of the body for the muscular strength and endurance training session. However, if you are beginning the training program, *always* start with shorter sessions and gradually build up to the longer training periods.

Specific training guidelines follow in Chapter 3 for flexibility, Chapter 4 for cardiorespiratory fitness, Chapter 5 for muscular strength and endurance, and Chapter 7 for modifying your body composition.

OTHER CONSIDERATIONS

In addition to the training principles and guidelines, there are other factors to consider before beginning your exercise program. These include your warm-up, cool-down, attire, mode of exercise, environment, nutrition, and rest. Additionally, misconceptions regarding exercise and exercises that may be contraindicated for you should be understood to ensure your safety and to maximize the results of your training program.

Warm-Up The .... nsists of an easy, whole-body activity prior to beginning the .... phases in the warm-up: cardiorespiratory, static stretching, ... arm-up should begin with a very low intensity cardiorespi......... he muscle and blood temperature to produce sweating but .... ue. Static stretching and light muscular endurance exercis......... mportant to warm up the specific muscles that you will use .... rior to activity not only prepares the body for participation

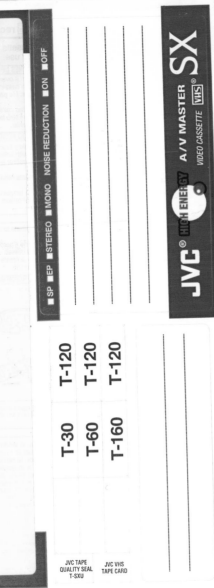

.... mplies a gradual tapering of activity. A good rule of thumb .... evel until your heart rate is below 100 beats per minute. .... ooling of the blood in the lower extremities. Static stretch......... process; it helps to reduce delayed localized soreness and

.... activity, the best attire for training usually consists of .... good pair of shoes, and an identification bracelet or tag. .... east one-half size larger than your everyday shoes in order .... toe and foot expansion, which occurs during impact with .... a medical alert tag should be worn if you have medical .... to in the event you are unable to communicate. Dress so .... mmer or become overexposed during the winter. During .... the head, ears, face, fingers, toes, and genitals. Layering .... l during the winter because you can remove outer layers .... ore prevent yourself from becoming overheated; it also .... der to avoid becoming chilled after perspiring. Listen to .... ngly. Protect yourself against foot and knee problems by .... aware that many activities require special equipment, such .... wear headphones when jogging or cycling, keep the vol......... ear traffic and safety signals.

.... e weight by exercising in rubber or plastic suits. This is a .... Wearing a rubber or plastic suit elevates your body tem......... ustion. Also, the weight loss from this practice is water .... u relieve your thirst by consuming fluids after the work......... suits when exercising.

.... ogram should consist of activities that you enjoy and that .... quate and safe training stimulus for cardiorespiratory fitness, flexibility, and muscular strength and endurance. For example, you may want to weight train on Mondays, Wednesdays, and Fridays and play full-court basketball on Tuesdays, Thursdays, and Saturdays. These activities, preceded by a warm-up and followed by a cool-down, would give you an adequate and safe training stimulus in each fitness component as long as you follow the SPORT FIT training guidelines. Chapters 3, 4, 5, and 7 have more specific information on training for flexibility, cardiorespiratory capacity, muscular strength, muscular endurance, and body composition. Remember, in order to develop or maintain fitness, you must regularly participate in a program that will develop all five components of fitness.

Environment.   Environmental conditions should be considered when structuring your program. These conditions include weather, terrain, altitude, pollution, type of facility, water temperature, and so on. Each of these factors will affect your performance.

In order to avoid dehydration on hot, humid days, drink plenty of fluids and avoid long training sessions where water may not be available. During the training session, drink fluids approximately every 20 minutes and immediately following the workout. Light-colored clothing will reflect some of the heat, keeping you cooler. Also, the time of day in which you train is especially important during the summer. Training in the early morning offers the advantage of cooler temperatures, while the evening hours are normally less humid. However, when training outdoors during low-light hours, be sure to wear reflective clothing or tape to alert motorists of your presence.

The main problems related to training in cold weather are frostbite and hypothermia. Frostbite normally occurs on the fingers, toes, penis, nose, and ears. To avoid frostbite of these areas, dress warmly. You can prevent hypothermia best by dressing warmly and by avoiding extremely low temperatures. Wearing dark clothing absorbs some of the sun's heat.

Environmental pollution is often a problem when training in urban areas. Exercising in high pollutant levels may lead to impaired lung function and decreased work capacity. In addition, the toxicity of environmental pollutants is increased during vigorous exercise due to greater air exchange in the lungs. If you live in a polluted area, it is best to train in the early morning or late evening when the pollutant levels are generally lower. The highest pollutant levels usually occur between 12 noon and 6 P.M. In addition, you should avoid jogging on roads with heavy traffic or near industrial factories. Dust may also be a problem; try to avoid areas with loose topsoil if the weather conditions have been dry and windy.

As the altitude increases, the partial pressure of oxygen decreases, thereby increasing the stress placed on the cardiorespiratory system during vigorous exercise. The human body normally adapts to this stress within 90 days by increasing the hemoglobin levels, which in turn increase the blood's oxygen-carrying capacity.

Nutrition.   The results you obtain from your training program also depend upon your diet. You should not attempt to participate in a training program without providing your body the essential nutrients. Proper nutrition contributes to the functioning of all bodily processes.

Unfortunately, much false information exists concerning diet and nutrition. Before depriving your body of nutrients by engaging in a fasting or weight-loss program, take time to read the information in Chapters 6 and 7 of this book.

Rest.   In addition to adequate exercise and nutrition, the body must receive enough rest in order to gain or maintain fitness. The body is able to withstand some abuse in regard to exercise, diet, and rest; however, abuse on a regular basis will lead to bad health. Give your body the rest it needs. On the average, people require six to nine hours of sleep a night.

MISCONCEPTIONS ABOUT EXERCISE

There are many misconceptions regarding exercise. One of these—the wearing of rubber or plastic suits—has already been discussed in the section on attire. Another misconception concerns gravity-inversion devices. Many fitness facilities offer devices that enable their members to hang upside down. These devices are supposed to increase flexibility, retard the aging process, reduce blood pressure, improve circulation, relieve back pain, and provide relaxation. Some facilities also recommend performing exercises while inverted on these devices. The physiological effects of head-down tilts of 130 degrees or less below the horizontal are well documented. However, there is little research available on head-down tilts of 180 degrees. A recent study indicates that head tilts of 180 degrees significantly increase the blood pressure of normal young adults. Therefore, it may be dangerous for hypertensive or borderline-hypertensive individuals to use inversion devices. In addition, since blood pressure increases with exercise, you should not exercise on gravity-inversion devices until further research is completed.

CONTRAINDICATED EXERCISES

Some exercises may damage your musculoskeletal system or cause trauma to your spinal column. These exercises are referred to as *contraindicated exercises*. It is especially important to consider your specific limitations before performing exercises. What may be an excellent exercise for a fit person may be contraindicated for an elderly person or for someone with musculoskeletal limitations such as arthritis, deteriorating discs, or back problems in general. Some exercises that are often considered contraindicated include the following:

1. rotation or hyperextension of the neck (Figure 2.1)
2. arm circles, which dynamically stretch the shoulder joint (Figure 2.2)
3. side bends, which overextend the spine laterally (Figure 2.3)
4. side-to-side twists or bends at the waist or of the trunk (Figures 2.4 and 2.5)
5. hyperextension of the back (Figure 2.6)
6. over-the-head back-and-shoulder stretch (Figure 2.7)
7. hamstring stretches that bend the body forward from the waist or twist from side to side (Figures 2.8 and 2.9)
8. traditional full sit-ups (Figure 2.10) and bent knee sit-ups (Figure 2.11), which put pressure on the vertebrae of the spine; crunches (Figure 2.12) are less likely to cause injury
9. hurdle stretch (Figure 2.13); Figure 2.14 shows an alternative stretch that inverts the knee

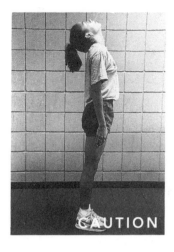

Figure 2.1

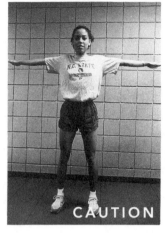

Figure 2.2

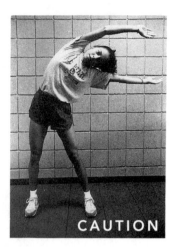

Figure 2.3

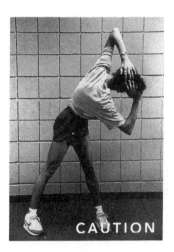

Figure 2.4

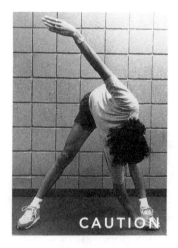

Figure 2.5

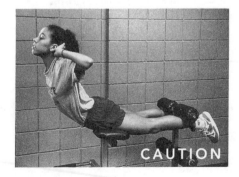

Figure 2.6

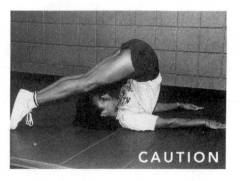

Figure 2.7

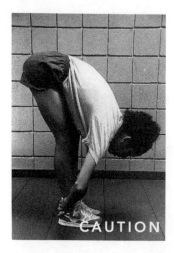

Figure 2.8

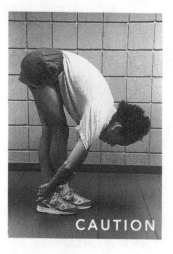

Figure 2.9

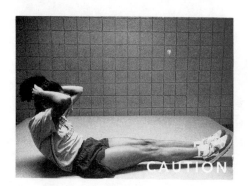

Figure 2.10

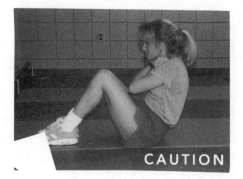

Figure 2.11

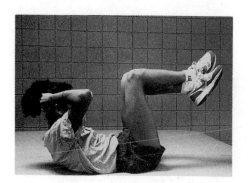

Figure 2.12

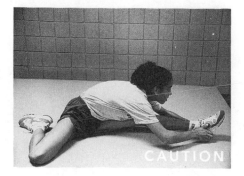

Figure 2.13

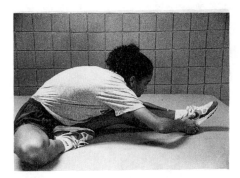

Figure 2.14

SUPPLEMENTARY READINGS

Allsen, P. E., J. M. Harrison, and B. Vance. *Fitness for Life: An Individualized Approach.* 5th ed. Madison, WI: Brown & Benchmark, 1993.

Harris, D. V., and J. A. Peterson. *Personal Fitness Guide.* Englewood, CO: Morton Publishing Company, 1988.

Hoeger, W. W. K. *Lifetime Physical Fitness.* 3d ed. Englewood, CO: Morton Publishing Company, 1992.

Lemarr, J. D. "Cardiorespiratory Responses to Inversion." *The Physician and Sportsmedicine.* Vol. 2, No. 2, November 1983.

Marley, W. P. *Health & Physical Fitness.* Dubuque, IA: Wm. C. Brown, 1988.

Mazzeo, K. A *Commitment to Fitness.* Englewood, CO: Morton Publishing Company, 1985.

CHAPTER 2 REVIEW QUESTIONS

1. Explain the following training principles:
   a. specificity:

   b. progression:

   c. overload:

   d. reversibility:

   e. training individuality:

2. Why is it important to warm up before the workout session?

3. Why is it important to cool down after the workout session?

4. What does *FIT* refer to in regard to a training program?

5. Describe the attire that should be worn during exercise.

6. How can you avoid becoming dehydrated when training on hot, humid days?

7. What are the main problems with training in cold weather, and how can you avoid them?

8. List at least two activities you enjoy that will help you develop the five components of fitness.

9. Why are proper nutrition and rest necessary for improving and maintaining your fitness level?

10. Why should you be concerned about exercising with gravity-inversion devices?

11. Why should you not attempt to lose weight by exercising in rubber or plastic suits?

12. Why are some exercises considered to be contraindicated?

CHAPTER
3

Flexibility

Flexibility is an important component of physical fitness but is frequently overlooked or ignored when planning fitness programs. The shape of the bones and cartilage in the joint, as well as the length of tendons, muscles, and ligaments crossing the joint, determine the degree of flexibility. The spectrum of flexibility ranges from that of extremely loose-jointed contortionists seen at the circus to that of arthritic patients with severely restricted ranges of movement. Adequate flexibility permits freedom of movement, contributes to the ease and efficiency of muscular effort, and helps to reduce susceptibility to some types of musculoskeletal problems and injuries. To increase the flexibility of a particular joint, safely stretch the specific tendons and muscles around that joint beyond their normal resting length. As a muscle reaches a fully stretched position, pain receptors in the muscle sense pain and trigger an involuntary protective response that causes the muscle to contract. This action is called the **stretch reflex.** Without such an automatic reaction, serious muscle or tendon injury could occur due to overstretching.

TYPES OF STRETCHING

There are basically two recommended types of stretching: static and proprioceptive neuromuscular facilitation. (A third type, dynamic stretching, consists of rapid bouncing or jerking movements that may lead to muscle and connective-tissue injury as well as muscle soreness. Therefore, most authorities do not recommend dynamic stretching for the development of flexibility.)

Static Stretching.   Static stretching, sometimes referred to as slow, sustained stretching, involves slowly stretching a muscle and holding it at greater than resting length for a short period of time. Muscles are gradually lengthened through the joint's complete range of motion, and the final position is held for six to ten seconds. Static stretching is the preferred method to improve flexibility in an exercise program because the chance of injury is less than with dynamic or proprioceptive neuromuscular stretching.

Proprioceptive Neuromuscular Facilitation.   Athletic teams and exercise classes often use proprioceptive neuromuscular facilitation (PNF). This type of stretching normally requires a partner, as well as more time, than the other methods of stretching. PNF involves a series of contractions and relaxations of the muscle fibers in the muscle group being stretched. Initially, your partner moves your particular limb partially through its range of movement (Figure 3.1).

At the angle at which movement is stopped, you should contract isometrically for a period of four to five seconds against the leverage your partner is applying. Upon completion of the isometric contraction, completely relax and allow your partner to move the limb to a greater angle but without causing you discomfort (Figure 3.2). **Always terminate a stretching exercise before feeling discomfort.**

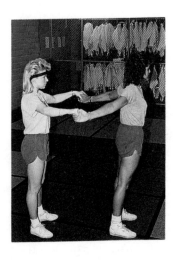

Figure 3.1

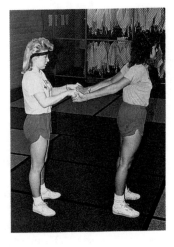

Figure 3.2

FLEXIBILITY TRAINING CONSIDERATIONS

Safety Considerations.   A circulatory warm-up should precede stretching exercises for flexibility. This includes easy, whole-body activity for four to six minutes. This activity elevates the heart rate and respiration rate, and increases the temperature of the muscles to help avoid injury during stretching.

Avoid forward flexion of the spine when stretching. The spine is a flexible column of vertebrae stacked on top of each other. Forward flexion causes the front border of the cushioning discs between the vertebrae to compress. This pressure may cause ruptured discs, especially if the forward flexion includes a twisting motion. Hyperextension of the spine, such as in back arches, can also lead to severe back pain by increasing the pressure on the discs.

Also avoid locking or hyperextending any joint when stretching. It is important to keep the joints slightly flexed in order to guard against tearing ligaments or connective tissue. Never force a movement that causes discomfort.

Specificity of Joint Mobility.   Flexibility is specific. You may possess a high degree of flexibility in some joints of the body and poor flexibility in others. Extensive and prolonged participation in a particular activity will result in development of flexibility only in those joints in which you constantly use the full range of motion while performing that activity.

Factors Influencing Flexibility. Flexibility depends upon several factors, such as mechanical limitations, activity levels, training techniques, posture, and age. Mechanical limitations include such things as natural or unnatural bone formation, fat deposits, and muscle mass, all of which set definite limits on the range of motion in some joints. Unnatural bone formations include calcium deposits and bone spurs. Also, the massive bulk of intervening muscle or fat tissue in heavily muscled or obese individuals may limit flexion of the elbow and knee.

People who are physically inactive generally tend to be less flexible than active people. This is partially due to the fact that not only muscles but also connective tissue, such as tendons and ligaments, tend to shorten through disuse.

Progressive-resistance exercises, such as weight training, are sometimes blamed for decreases in flexibility. However, this is a false assertion. Muscle-boundness, the term for individuals with bulging muscles and a lack of flexibility, is caused by poor training techniques. In order to avoid muscle-boundness, you should perform exercises through the full range of motion, exercise the antagonist (opposite) muscle group, and include stretching in your warm-up and cool-down routines.

Faulty posture can also influence flexibility by causing some muscles to shorten. For example, if you constantly assume a round-shouldered, slouched posture, gradual shortening of the pectoral muscles of the chest will occur. This, in turn, will adversely affect shoulder flexibility.

Age and sex are other factors influencing flexibility. As children develop, they tend to increase in flexibility until adolescence. During the adolescent years, a gradual loss of joint flexibility begins that continues throughout adult life. A proper flexibility program can lessen this reduction.

Flexibility and Lower-Back Pain. Millions of Americans suffer from chronic lower-back pain due primarily to weak abdominal and hip-flexor muscles in conjunction with poor flexibility of the lower-back and hip-extensor muscles. The weak abdominal muscles are unable to exert sufficient tension to prevent the pelvis from tilting forward and downward. This causes excessive arching in the lower back and slight displacement of the vertebrae. The resulting pressure on adjacent nerves causes chronic pain in the lower area of the back. You can voluntarily exaggerate the lower back (lumbar) curvature by tilting the pelvis forward and downward to experience similar discomfort.

The solution to this problem of lower-back pain lies in developing and then maintaining adequate abdominal and hip-flexor muscle strength combined with increased flexibility of the hip extensors and the lower back (gluteus maximus and hamstrings). Promptly seek medical attention when more serious causes of back pain—such as arthritis, kidney disease, and spinal defects—are suspected. Chapter 5 provides additional information on strengthening the abdominals and hip flexors.

The sit-and-reach test is often used to measure the flexibility of the lower back and hip extensors. This test consists of sitting on the floor with legs together and extended so that the soles of the feet are flat against the side of the box, with the buttocks, spine, and back of the head against the wall as shown in Figure 3.3. Your arms should be extended and your shoulders rounded while your partner slides the yardstick forward or backward to adjust the end of the yardstick to the tips of your fingers. With the yardstick secure in the adjusted position, bend at the waist and slowly slide your fingers along the yardstick as far as possible, as shown in Figure 3.4, using static stretching. Your partner will read your score to the nearest quarter-inch on the yardstick. Norms for college students, ages 17 to 25, are listed in Table 3.1.

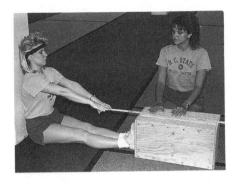

Figure 3.3

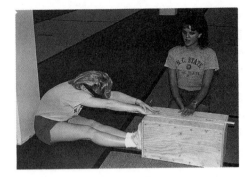

Figure 3.4

Table 3.1   Norms for the sit-and-reach.

PERCENTILE	FEMALES	MALES
99	21.5	21.5
95	19.0	19.25
90	18.0	18.0
85	17.5	17.25
80	17.0	17.0
75	16.5	16.5
70	16.0	16.0
65	15.5	15.5
60	15.0	15.0
55	14.5	14.5
50	14.25	14.25
45	14.0	14.0
40	13.5	13.75
35	13.25	13.25
30	13.0	13.0
25	12.0	12.0
20	11.5	11.5
15	11.0	10.75
10	10.0	9.75
05	8.0	9.0

FLEXIBILITY TRAINING GUIDELINES

Be sure to incorporate the following guidelines into your flexibility program.

1. Begin the flexibility routine with an easy whole-body activity—such as rope skipping, running in place, or other cardiorespiratory exercise—to raise your body temperature. Most experts believe that elevating body temperature through exercise tends to increase the pliability of connective tissue such as tendons and thus provides greater potential for increased flexibility and less chance of injury.

2. Never hyperextend, or hyperflex, or lock any joint during stretching exercises. Do not force body parts beyond their range of motion. Be especially careful during PNF stretching, where this can easily occur. Always stretch your muscles slowly and gently.

3. A minimum of five stretch repetitions should be performed for each exercise. Static stretch repetitions should be held in the stretch position for six to ten seconds, and the PNF stretch should be held for four to five seconds.

4. Be very careful when performing stretching exercises involving the spinal column. Avoid extreme movements of the trunk and neck.

5. Remember, flexibility is specific to each joint. Therefore, perform stretching exercises for each muscle group or joint in which you want to increase flexibility.

6. Exercises that do not create **stretch demand**—that is, muscle lengthening beyond normal—will not improve flexibility.

7. Stretching exercises must be performed regularly. The fitness adage "Use it or lose it" applies as much to flexibility as it does to other components of fitness.

8. Avoid exercises that may be contraindicated for you. Review Chapter 2.

STRETCHING EXERCISES

This section discusses a number of stretching exercises. Use either of the two recommended methods of stretching with these exercises to develop your personal stretching program.

Lateral Head Tilt

Purpose: To stretch the neck flexors and extensors, and ligaments of the cervical spine.

Starting position (Figure 3.5): Keep your head upright and relaxed.

Movement (Figure 3.6): Slowly and gently tilt your head laterally. Hold for six to ten seconds. Return to starting position and repeat several times to each side.

Precaution: Do not hyperextend or rotate the neck, as this can cause damage to the cervical discs.

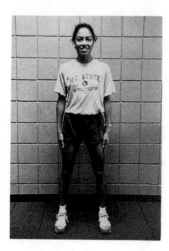

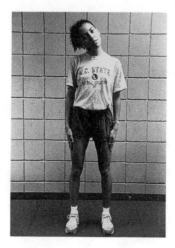

Figure 3.5

Figure 3.6

Shoulder Stretches

Purpose: To stretch the shoulders, chest, and upper back.

Starting position (Figure 3.7): Extend your arms overhead and place your palms together.

Movement: Stretch your arms upward and slightly backward. Breathe in as you stretch upward, holding the stretch six to ten seconds.

Starting position (Figure 3.8): Place your right arm across your chest, with your left hand supporting your right elbow.

Movement: With your left hand, gently pull your right elbow toward your left shoulder. Hold the stretch for six to ten seconds. Then repeat the stretch on the opposite side.

Starting position (Figure 3.9): Raise your arms overhead, with both elbows bent. Hold the elbow of your left arm behind your head with your right hand.

Movement: Gently pull your elbow downward behind your head. Hold the stretch for six to ten seconds. Repeat the exercise on the opposite side.

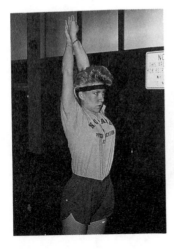

Figure 3.7

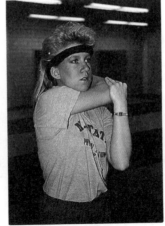

Figure 3.8

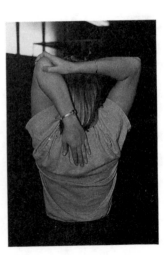

Figure 3.9

Back Stretches

Purpose: To stretch the latissimus dorsi, a large muscle of the back that extends from the lower spine and attaches to the upper arm.

Starting position (Figure 3.10): Position your right arm diagonally across your face, with your left hand supporting your right elbow.

Movement (Figure 3.11): With your hand, gently pull your right elbow diagonally across and in front of your face. Hold the stretch for six to ten seconds. Repeat the stretch on the opposite side.

Starting position (Figure 3.12): Lie flat on the floor in a supine position.

Movement (Figure 3.13): Slowly curl both knees toward your head into a fetal position, clasp arm around lower legs just below your knees, and hold this position for six to ten seconds.

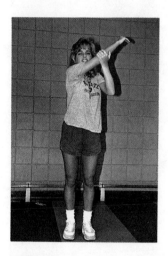

Figure 3.10

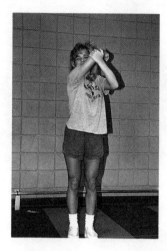

Figure 3.11

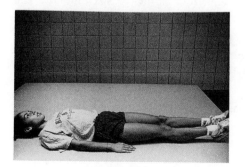

Figure 3.12

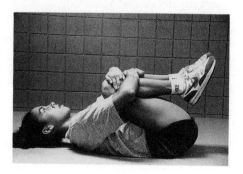

Figure 3.13

Chest-and-Shoulder Stretch

Purpose: To stretch the chest and front of the shoulders.

Starting position (Figure 3.14):   Stand with your feet parallel to the wall with your feet approximately six inches from the wall. Raise your right arm up with the elbow bent at a right angle and place your right hand and forearm against the wall.

Movement (Figure 3.15):   With your hand and forearm placed on wall, rotate your body backward around the shoulder joint. Keep your hand and forearm stationary on the wall during the movement in order to apply the stretch. Repeat the sequence on the other side.

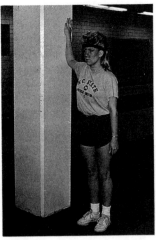

Figure 3.14

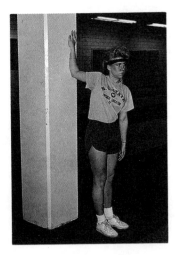

Figure 3.15

Chest-and-Shoulder Stretch

Purpose: To stretch the chest and front of the shoulders.

Starting position (Figure 3.16):   In a standing position, extend both arms at the elbow and move them slightly behind your body at shoulder height. Your partner grasps your arms just above the wrists.

Movement (Figure 3.17):   Your partner slowly brings your arms closer together until tightness is felt in your chest and shoulders. Your partner then holds the angle, and you contract isometrically for five seconds and then relax. Terminate before feeling mild discomfort.

Precaution: This is a PNF stretch that swim teams often use. This stretch is contraindicated for many individuals. Remember, always terminate stretching before you feel discomfort.

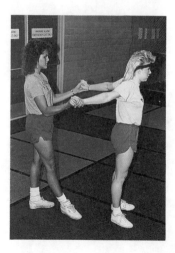

Figure 3.16

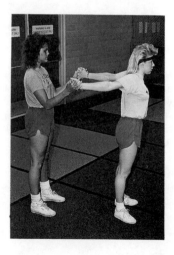

Figure 3.17

Side Stretch

Purpose: To stretch the lateral (side) portions of the trunk.

Starting position (Figure 3.18):   Start with your feet approximately shoulder-width apart and one arm raised over your head. Place the hand of the other arm on the upper thigh and support the side to which you are leaning.

Movement (Figure 3.19):   Reach high with your arm and slightly lean to the opposite side. Return to the starting position and repeat the movement on the opposite side.

Precaution: Avoid rotating your torso as you go through the movement. Do not move the spine farther than 20 degrees to the side from the vertical position.

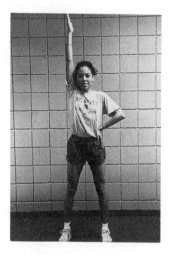

Figure 3.18

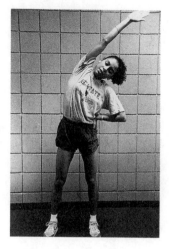

Figure 3.19

Hip, Thigh, and Ankle Stretch

Purpose: To stretch the front of the hips, upper legs, and lower legs.

Starting position (Figure 3.20):   Stand upright, facing a wall, with your weight on your right foot. Brace your right hand against the wall to maintain your balance. Bend your left knee and grasp your lower leg slightly above the ankle with your left hand. Extend your hip forward to stretch the front of the hip and upper leg. Keep your spine erect.

Movement (Figure 3.21):   Slowly pull your left ankle upward and rearward away from your left buttock and slightly extend the hip forward. Hold this position and contract by attempting to extend your knee. Hold the isometric contraction for four to five seconds. Relax. Repeat the movement. Relax. Terminate this sequence before you feel mild discomfort. Repeat the exercise on the opposite side. Note that this exercise uses the PNF method.

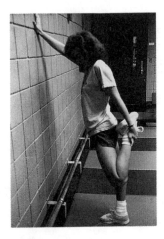

Figure 3.20

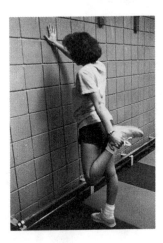

Figure 3.21

Hamstring Stretch

Purpose: To stretch the back of the thighs (hamstrings).

Starting position: Seated on the floor, slightly separate your feet, with the backs of your legs flat against the floor.

Movement (Figure 3.22):   While keeping your spine straight, slowly reach forward toward your toes. Hold the stretch for six to ten seconds.

Hip Extensor Stretch

Purpose: To stretch the hip extensors (buttocks).

Starting position: Begin in a supine position, with your hands at your sides and feet together.

Movement (Figure 3.23): Slowly draw one knee up toward your chest. Grasp your hands behind this knee and slowly draw it further toward your chest. Hold the stretch for six to ten seconds. Keep your opposite leg flat on the mat. Relax and return to the starting position. Repeat on the opposite side.

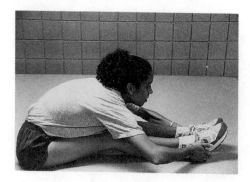

Figure 3.22

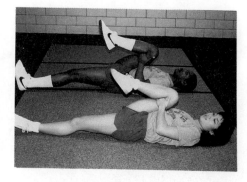

Figure 3.23

Inner-Thigh-and-Groin Stretch

Purpose: To stretch the inner thighs and the groin area.

Starting position: Stand upright with your feet approximately three feet apart.

Movement (Figure 3.24): Slide your right leg sideways approximately one foot, bend your right knee, and shift your body weight toward the right in trying to sit over your right ankle while keeping your left leg straight. Hold the stretch for six to ten seconds. Repeat the sequence on the opposite side.

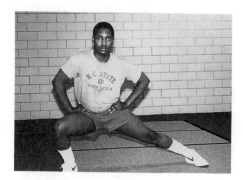

Figure 3.24

Calf Stretch

Purpose: To stretch the back of the lower legs.

Starting position (Figure 3.25): Begin in an inclined body position facing a wall, with your hands against the wall. Slightly separate and stagger your feet, with the foot closest to the wall approximately 18 inches away from the wall. Your leg nearer to the wall should be bent at the knee. Place the heels of both feet flat on the floor.

Movement (Figure 3.26): Keep your body straight, in diagonal alignment to the wall. Bend your arms at the elbows, allowing your body to lean forward while keeping your heels flat on the floor. Hold this stretch for six to ten seconds.

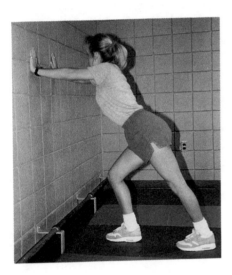

Figure 3.25

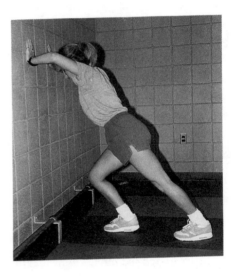

Figure 3.26

Achilles Stretch

Purpose: To stretch the Achilles tendons.

Starting position (Figure 3.25): Just as for the calf stretch, begin in an inclined body position with your hands against a wall, your feet slightly separated and staggered with the front foot approximately 18 inches away from the wall. Your leg closer to the wall is bent at the knee. Keep the heels of both feet flat on the floor.

Movement (Figures 3.26, 3.27): Keep your body straight, in diagonal alignment to the wall. Bend your arms at the elbows, allowing your body to lean forward, and keep your heels flat on the floor. Bend the knee of your rear leg. Hold the stretch for six to ten seconds.

Remember, flexibility is an important component of fitness. Now is the time to incorporate flexibility into your fitness program.

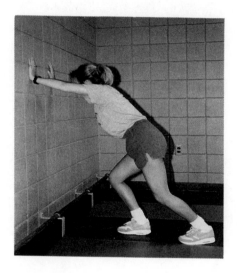

Figure 3.27

SUPPLEMENTARY READINGS

American College of Obstetricians and Gynecologists. *Guidelines for Women Who Exercise.* Washington, DC: ACOG, 1986.

Branner, T. *The Safe Exercise Handbook.* Dubuque, IA: Kendall/Hunt, 1993.

Chastain, S. M. *Aerobics: A Guide for Participants.* 2d ed. Dubuque, IA: Kendall/Hunt, 1993.

Corbin, C. B., and R. Lindsey. *Concepts of Physical Fitness with Laboratories.* 8th ed. Madison, WI: Brown & Benchmark, 1994.

DeVries, H. A., and T. J. Housh. *Physiology of Exercise for Physical Education, Athletics and Exercise Science.* 5th ed. Madison, WI: Brown & Benchmark, 1994.

Hoeger, W. W. K. *Fitness and Wellness.* 2d ed. Englewood, CO: Morton Publishing, 1993.

CHAPTER 3 REVIEW QUESTIONS

1. List the two recommended types of stretching described in this chapter.

    a.

    b.

2. Which type of stretching is most highly recommended?

3. List five factors that influence flexibility.

    a.

    b.

    c.

    d.

    e.

4. What is believed to be the cause of chronic lower-back pain for most Americans?

5. How can you prevent chronic lower-back pain?

6. What test can you use to measure the flexibility of the lower back and hip extensors?

7. Briefly summarize the flexibility training guidelines.

CHAPTER

4

Cardiorespiratory Fitness

Most physical fitness experts consider cardiorespiratory (CR) fitness to be the most important component of physical fitness. Cardiorespiratory fitness refers to the efficiency of the body in transporting and utilizing oxygen.

The organs associated with the intake, delivery, and utilization of oxygen are the heart and lungs—hence the term *cardio* (heart) *respiratory* (breathing). Oxygen is the catalyst that initiates the burning of calories to produce energy, a process known as **oxidation.** During exercise, an increase in energy expenditure calls for a similar increase in the amount of oxygen required for oxidation to take place. When your cardiorespiratory system cannot meet the increased demand for oxygen during heightened physical activity, you need to reduce the intensity of the activity in order to balance the amount of oxygen required and the amount that can be delivered.

Since we live in an environment with an unlimited supply of oxygen, the problem of obtaining enough oxygen is not an external one, but rather an internal one. The ability of the cardiorespiratory system to process oxygen can be so severely limited in some unconditioned people that even slight increases in energy demands, like climbing a flight of stairs, can cause both heart and respiration rates to rise significantly.

TRAINING GUIDELINES FOR CARDIORESPIRATORY FITNESS

Certain factors concerning the quality and quantity of training should be considered in the development and maintenance of cardiorespiratory fitness. These include the mode, frequency, intensity, and time (duration) (FIT) of exercise. In addition, you should consider your physical limitations.

Mode.   Participation in a training program that includes individual or group aerobic activities can help you attain cardiorespiratory fitness. Aerobic activities are those that

35

are rhythmic in nature, can be sustained for an extended period of time, and involve large-muscle groups. Aerobic activities include aerobics, jogging, running, swimming, fitness walking, cycling, rowing, speed skating, rope skipping, ultimate frisbee, water aerobics, basketball, soccer, and many other sustained-movement activities.

You should choose enjoyable but vigorous activities that provide a training stimulus. Using a variety of activities in your program tends to relieve boredom, reduce injuries caused from overuse, and produce overall fitness. After you have chosen aerobic activities to use in your training program, you will need to apply the FIT guidelines to improve your cardiorespiratory fitness. Recall that *FIT* refers to frequency, intensity, and time.

Frequency.   In order to achieve and maintain cardiorespiratory fitness, you must exercise on a regular basis. Generally, *training three to five days per week is recommended.* Training less than three days per week appears to be inadequate for gains in cardiorespiratory fitness, while training more than five days per week results in greater incidence of injury. After reaching a desired level of fitness, you can maintain that approximate level by training twice per week. Upon cessation of a training program, a significant reduction in working capacity begins to occur after two weeks.

Weight-bearing activities—such as running and jumping—result in a higher incidence of injury than do non-weight-bearing activities—such as swimming and cycling—due to the amount of stress generated on the joints of the ankles, knees, and hips. Using a variety of activities in a cardiorespiratory program tends to reduce injuries caused by overuse.

Intensity.   For healthy young adults the heart rate is a good indicator of the intensity of an activity. The American College of Sports Medicine recommends that the intensity of the activity be vigorous enough to increase the heart rate to 60 to 90 percent of the **maximum heart rate reserve.** This range is referred to as the **target heart rate zone.** Maximum heart rate reserve represents the difference between the **R**esting **H**eart **R**ate (RHR) and the **M**aximum **H**eart **R**ate (MHR), added to the resting heart rate.

Target heart rate lower limit = .6(MHR – RHR) + RHR

Target heart rate upper limit = .9(MHR – RHR) + RHR

The best method of determining the maximum heart rate is to perform a graded-exercise stress test on a treadmill. However, due to the expense of the graded-exercise stress test, the maximum heart rate for young, healthy adults is often estimated by subtracting their ages from (the index number of) 220. For example, if you are 18 years old, 202 would be an estimate of your maximum heart rate (220 – 18 = 202). The maximum heart rate decreases for most individuals at the rate of 1.1 beats per year after the age of 25.

Example: Joe is a 20-year-old healthy adult male who has a maximum heart rate of 200 beats per minute (bpm) and a resting heart rate of 72 bpm. Therefore, his target heart rate zone would be:

Lower limit = .6(200 – 72) + 72 = 148.8 bpm

Upper limit = .9(200 – 72) + 72 = 187.2 bpm

In order to gain or maintain cardiorespiratory fitness, Joe should monitor his heart rate as he trains and vary the intensity of his activity in order to ensure that he is within the target heart rate zone.

Figure your target heart rate zone:

Lower limit = .6(____ – ____) + ____ = ____ bpm

Upper limit = .9(____ – ____) + ____ = ____ bpm

You should train near the lower limit of the target heart rate zone, 60 percent of MHR, when beginning a program. *Exercise does not have to be unbearable or painful in order to obtain a reasonable level of cardiorespiratory fitness.* Training at the lower limit of the target heart rate zone represents moderately intense activity that can be continued for an extended period of time with little discomfort. Once the benefits of training begin to occur, you can safely increase your training intensity to higher levels within the target heart rate zone.

Time (Duration). *The training session should be 20 to 60 minutes of continuous aerobic activity, with 20 to 30 minutes being a very reasonable goal.* For the greatest improvement per unit of exercise time, 30 minutes appears to be best. Generally, the greater the intensity, the shorter the duration, and vice versa.

Precautions. *All individuals over 35, regardless of health status, should complete a physical examination before beginning a training program.* Also, if you have any medical problems, have a complete medical exam regardless of your age.

Participation in a fitness program can benefit almost everyone. Once you have identified your physical limitations, you should be able to use the information presented in this textbook to plan a vigorous and enjoyable program that can also be therapeutic.

Before beginning a training session, warm up the muscle groups and joints that will be involved in the workout. Begin the exercise slowly, and then increase the pace until reaching the desired target heart rate. Monitor the heart rate periodically to determine if the pace is too fast or too slow. After a few training sessions, you will be able to feel when you reach the target heart rate. In order to reduce the chance of injury and needless fatigue, be sure to perform the activity with proper form and technique.

Do not overtrain! Initially, the training progression should be slow. If just beginning a program, train every other day. Let the body have the time it needs for recovery by alternating hard and easy days. After the muscles and tendons have toughened and become accustomed to the training routine, you can increase the progression. Remember, using a variety of activities helps prevent boredom as well as injuries from overuse.

Do not attempt to exercise through persistent pain. If localized pain increases during exercise, stop the workout. If you experience shortness of breath, chest pain, dizziness, or nausea, terminate the exercise and consult a physician.

Continue to move at the end of the training session in order to prevent the blood from pooling in the working muscles. Monitor the heart to determine the recovery rate during the first few minutes after exercising. The rate of recovery will be faster as your fitness level improves. At the end of the workout, cool down slowly and stretch the muscles used. The muscles are warmest at this time, and you can attain a significant increase in flexibility.

ASSESSING CARDIORESPIRATORY FITNESS

The most accurate way to assess cardiorespiratory fitness is to measure your maximum oxygen uptake, VO_2max, by using a graded-exercise stress test on a treadmill. VO_2max is the maximal rate at which oxygen can be taken up, distributed, and used by the body in the performance of exercise that utilizes large-muscle groups. Norms for maximal oxygen uptake are listed in Table 4.1. However, since the graded-exercise test is expensive and time-consuming, it generally is not used for most healthy adults. More practical but less accurate tests include the step test, a one-mile walk, and the 1.5-mile run. College fitness classes often use these measures to determine cardiorespiratory fitness. Tables 1.1 and 1.2 in Chapter 1 provide norms for the step test; Table 4.2 provides norms for the 1.5-mile run.

The following formula[*] can be used to predict your VO_2max for the one-mile walk. After an adequate warm-up, complete a one-mile walk on a measured track as fast as you can and record the elapsed time. Calculate your heart rate in beats per minute at the end of the walk. Applying this information to the following formula allows you to calculate your VO_2max.

$$VO_2max = \quad 6.9652$$

$$+ \quad (0.0091 \times body\ weight)$$
$$- \quad (0.02576 \times age)$$
$$+ \quad (0.5955 \times gender)$$
$$- \quad (0.2240 \times time)$$
$$- \quad (0.0115 \times HR)$$
$$\times \quad [1,000 \div (body\ weight/2.2046)]$$

where: body weight = weight in pounds
gender = 0 for females; 1 for males
time = time to complete one-mile walk in minutes
HR = heart rate in beats/minute at end of walk

For example, if Jennie is 25 years old, weighs 130 pounds, and can walk a mile in 12.5 minutes with an ending HR of 128 beats/minute, her VO_2max is calculated as follows:

$$VO_2max = \quad 6.9652$$

$$+ \quad (0.0091 \times 130)$$
$$- \quad (0.0257 \times 25)$$
$$+ \quad (0.5955 \times 0)$$
$$- \quad (0.2240 \times 12.5)$$
$$- \quad (0.0115 \times 128)$$
$$\times \quad [1,000 \div (130/2.2046)]$$

$$\overline{}$$

54.84 ml/kg/min

Using the norms for VO_2max found in Table 4.1, this student is classified as being in the "excellent" category for cardiorespiratory fitness.

Since resting heart rate decreases with improvement of cardiorespiratory fitness, you

[*]derived by George, Vehrs, Allsen, Fellingham, and Fisher.

Table 4.1 VO$_2$max norms based on age and gender.

AGE	EXCELLENT	VERY GOOD	GOOD	AVERAGE	FAIR	POOR	VERY POOR
MAXIMAL OXYGEN CONSUMPTION (ML/KG/MIN)							
Women							
20–29	53	47–52	43–51	37–42	33–36	27–32	26
30–39	47	44–46	38–43	34–37	30–33	25–29	24
40–49	42	38–41	34–37	30–33	26–29	22–25	21
50–59	37	34–36	30–33	26–29	23–25	19–22	18
60–69	31	28–30	25–27	22–24	19–21	16–18	15
70+	26	24–25	21–23	18–20	15–17	13–14	12
Men							
20–29	64	56–63	51–55	45–50	38–44	32–37	31
30–39	57	52–56	46–51	41–45	35–40	29–34	28
40–49	53	47–51	42–45	37–41	32–36	27–31	26
50–59	47	42–46	37–41	33–36	28–32	24–27	23
60–69	42	37–42	33–36	28–33	25–27	21–24	20
70+	36	32–35	28–31	25–27	22–24	18–21	17

Adapted from Shrantz, E., and Reibold, R. C. "Aerobic fitness norms for males and females aged 6 to 75 years: A review." *Aviation, Space, and Environmental Medicine* 61: 3–11, 1990.

Table 4.2 Norms for the 1.5-mile run test.

FITNESS CATEGORY	GENDER	TIME AGE 17–25	TIME AGE 26–35
Superior	Males	8:30	9:30
	Females	10:30	11:30
Excellent	Males	8:30–9:29	9:30–10:29
	Females	10:30–11:49	11:30–12:49
Good	Males	9:30–10:29	10:30–11:29
	Females	11:50–13:09	12:50–14:09
Moderate	Males	10:30–11:29	11:30–12:29
	Females	13:10–14:29	14:10–15:29
Fair	Males	11:30–12:29	12:30–13:29
	Females	14:30–15:49	15:30–16:49
Poor	Males	>12:20	>13:29
	Females	>15:49	>16:49

Note: Before taking this running test, it is highly recommended that the student or individual be "moderately fit." Sedentary people should first start an exercise program and slowly build up to 20 minutes of running, 3 days per week, before taking this test.

From Draper, D. O., and Jones, G. L. "The 1.5 mile run revisited—An update in women's times." *JOPERD*, 78–80, September 1990.

Table 4.3 YMCA norms for resting heart rate (beats/min).

AGE (YR)	18–25		26–35		36–45		46–55		56–65		>65	
GENDER	M	F	M	F	M	F	M	F	M	F	M	F
Excellent	49–55	54–60	49–54	54–59	50–56	54–59	50–57	54–60	51–56	54–59	50–55	54–59
Good	57–61	61–65	57–61	60–64	60–62	62–64	59–63	61–65	59–61	61–64	58–61	60–64
Above average	63–65	66–69	62–65	66–68	64–66	66–69	64–67	66–69	64–67	67–69	62–65	66–68
Average	67–69	70–73	66–70	69–71	68–70	70–72	68–71	70–73	68–71	71–73	66–69	70–72
Below average	71–73	74–78	72–74	72–76	73–76	74–78	73–76	74–77	72–75	75–77	70–73	73–76
Poor	76–81	80–84	77–81	78–82	77–82	79–82	79–83	78–84	76–81	79–81	75–79	79–84
Very poor	84–95	86–100	84–94	84–94	86–96	84–92	85–97	85–96	84–94	85–96	83–98	88–96

Adapted from *Y's Way to Fitness* (3rd ed.). Reprinted with permission from the YMCA of the USA.

may wonder why the resting pulse is not commonly used as a measure of cardiorespiratory fitness. The resting pulse is subject to fluctuations caused by a number of variables, including body temperature, environmental temperature and humidity, anxiety and emotional stress, degree of hydration, food intake, and medication. Unless these factors are controlled, resting heart rate as a measure of cardiorespiratory fitness is often unreliable and misleading. Norms for the resting heart rate are found in Table 4.3.

MONITORING THE HEART RATE

You can monitor your heart rate best at those points on the body where arteries lie close to the skin surface. The heart rate or pulse is normally taken at the base of the thumb joint on the inside of the wrist (radial artery pulse) and in the groove to the side of the Adam's apple (carotid artery pulse). It is best to take your carotid pulse on the same side of the body as the hand that monitors the pulse in order to avoid restriction of blood flow. Important points to remember when monitoring the pulse are to use your fingers, not your thumb, and not to press too firmly against the artery, especially the carotid artery. Pressing too firmly may shut off the blood supply. Also, pressing too firmly may cause the baroreceptors in the carotid arteries to send messages to the brain that will cause the heart to slow its rate of beating. This may give inaccurate results.

In counting the pulse rate, the longer the count is taken, the more accurate it will be. When measuring the resting heart rate, a long count is desirable. However, a long count will not accurately reflect immediate postexercise heart rate since the pulse rate begins to drop from the level attained in exercise immediately following cessation of exercise. Therefore, a short count is advisable when taking the immediate postexercise heart rate. The discrepancy between the immediate postexercise rate and the rate one or two minutes later can be as much as 30 beats. In order to obtain an immediate postexercise heart rate that is indicative of heart rate attained during exercise, a short count started immediately after completion of exercise is necessary. When starting an exercise program, you can monitor your intensity by stopping and taking your pulse rate several times during your workout. One popular method is to count the heart rate for 10 seconds and multiply by six to determine the rate per minute. Another is to count for six seconds and attach a zero to the end of the number of beats counted. For example, if you counted 16 beats in 10 seconds, attach a zero and you obtain 160 beats per minute. On the step-test pulse recovery used in this textbook, the count is for 15 seconds. Therefore, the count is multiplied by four to obtain the rate per minute. The pulse rate is always recorded as the number of heartbeats per minute.

TRAINING EFFECTS OF A CARDIORESPIRATORY FITNESS PROGRAM

When the body receives a cardiorespiratory training stimulus on a regular basis, physiological changes begin to occur. The heart enlarges, becomes stronger, and is more efficient. The **stroke volume,** the amount of blood pumped out of the left ventricle with each beat, increases. The resting pulse decreases, as does the pulse rate for any given submaximal workload. Increased capillarization around the cells improves the oxygen diffusion at the cellular level. This accelerates the process of replenishing the cells with nutrients and removing metabolic wastes. Also, it improves the collateral circulation feeding the heart. This increases your chance of surviving a heart attack by providing alternate pathways for blood vessels around a blocked artery.

In addition, training enables the arteries to better maintain their elasticity, which in turn enables them to accommodate great pressures. Likewise, the number of red blood cells increases, providing more hemoglobin for transporting oxygen to the cells. Training also reduces low-density lipoproteins and increases high-density lipoproteins, affording increased protection against coronary heart disease.

Participating in a fitness program can help you to live a more productive life. Training can help maintain ideal body weight and help reduce stress. You will feel better and have more energy in your daily activities when you maintain a high level of fitness.

CARDIORESPIRATORY ACTIVITIES

As mentioned earlier in this chapter, cardiorespiratory activities are those activities that are rhythmic in nature, can be sustained for a long period of time, and use large-muscle groups in the body. In order to provide a cardiorespiratory training stimulus, these activities must meet the requirements of frequency, intensity, and time. The activities you choose to include in your training program should be enjoyable. If not, you may experience difficulty in staying with the program. To help monitor your heart beat, use the cardiorespiratory start sheet and the cardiorespiratory progress chart in Appendix B.

Jogging and Running. These activities have become extremely popular in the last 15 years. They provide an excellent training stimulus for cardiorespiratory gains and are easy to control with respect to frequency, intensity, and time. Jogging and running (Figure 4.1) require little equipment and give the individual a sense of freedom.

The disadvantage of jogging or running is the high incidence of injury. Injuries occur for many reasons, including the weight-bearing nature of the activities, poor anatomical structure in some individuals, improper training progression, and overuse. Common injuries include tendinitis, shin soreness or shin splints, blisters, stress fractures, foot and knee sprains, jogger's nipple, jogger's toe, muscle injuries and strains, chondromalacia patellae (runner's knee), and dehydration. You can avoid the majority of these injuries with proper foot support and clothing, adequate warm-up and cool-down, slow training progression, and staying within the training limitations of your anatomical structure. Research indicates that it is not necessary to run more than three miles five times a week in order to maintain a reasonable level of cardiorespiratory fitness. If you run more than this, you are probably

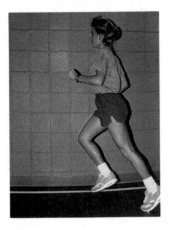

Figure 4.1

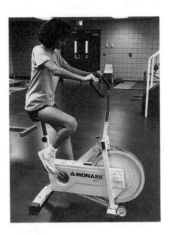

Figure 4.2

running for a reason other than general cardiorespiratory fitness. Appendix B provides you with a cardiorespiratory start sheet and a cardiorespiratory progress chart.

Cycling.   The number of cyclists has greatly increased during the last decade. This trend appears to be partly the result of the increasing popularity of triathlons, coupled with the high incidence of running and jogging injuries. Cycling allows you to tour the countryside while receiving an excellent cardiorespiratory training stimulus. Many people use a stationary bicycle (Figure 4.2) during inclement weather or in areas where traffic is hazardous.

The disadvantages of cycling include dogs, accidents, and the cost of cycling equipment. A common injury in cycling has been chondromalacia patellae, which is a softening of cartilage under the kneecap. However, you can normally prevent this injury by supplementing the cycling program with the leg extension exercise, using light resistance and moving through the last quarter of the range of motion to full knee extension. This exercise is discussed in more detail in Chapter 5.

Swimming.   Swimming (Figure 4.3) is a non-weight-bearing cardiorespiratory activity that is excellent when used either as a program in itself or to supplement other activities. Swimming provides a total-body workout using the resistance of water. You can use swimming to maintain cardiorespiratory fitness when resting from a hard workout in another activity or recuperating from an injury. Approximately 103 million people a year swim for rehabilitation, leisure, or competition.

There are over 218,000 master swimmers in the U. S. with the credo of fun, fitness, and competition. Members participate in a wide range of activities from noncompetitive lap swimming to international competition. US Swimming, Inc. is the national governing body for amateur competitive swimming in the United States.

Due to the non-weight-bearing and aquatic nature of the activity, swimming offers four advantages over most other activities. First, the cooling effect of the water helps maintain your body temperature closer to normal during exercise. Second, there is less trauma to the joints. The third advantage is that blood return to the heart through the veins is facilitated by the reduced effect of gravity. The last advantage involves the therapeutic nature of the

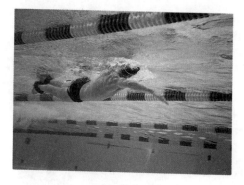

Figure 4.3

water in general and in treatment of injuries. In water, you are able to exercise through a full range of motion with minimal resistance, the buoyancy of the water providing support for the injured limb.

However, swimming also has its disadvantages. Swimming laps in a pool may become boring unless you periodically introduce variety into your training methods. In addition, eye irritation or injury may occur if you do not wear goggles or adjust them properly. Swimmer's ear can also be a problem if you allow moisture to remain in your ear canal.

Some methods of training for swimming consist of self-paced and strict intervals, long slow distance, over distance, Fartlek, negative split, progressive training, and a variety of water exercises. The use of kicking and pulling aids are also employed in most training. Example workout approximate time: 30 minutes.

Warm-Up:	Swim 300 yds. easily, changing strokes
Main Set:	Freestyle swim, 4×100 yds., with 15-second rest in lower THRZ
	Kick 250 yds., changing kicks
	Pull buoy 250 yds. freestyle
	Individual medleys, 4×100 yds., with 15-second rest in middle to upper THRZ
	35 pressouts (while hanging onto the side of the pool, fully extend elbows to straighten the arms and lift the body upward)
Cool-Down:	100 yds. easy swim
Total Distance:	1,700 yds.

Fitness Walking. Fitness walking is an enjoyable mode of exercise that you can participate in for most of your life. Walking places less stress on the joints than do jogging and running. Fitness walking requires proper form such as good posture, a heel–toe roll as the foot strikes the ground, and a vigorous arm swing. Fitness walkers can usually walk a mile in about 12 to 17 minutes. To walk year-round, many choose mall walking before stores open. Walking is ideal if you are obese, because there is less strain on your bones and joints than other weight-bearing aerobic activities. As with any form of cardiorespiratory activity, walking should be performed within the guidelines specified by the American College of Sports Medicine in regard to frequency, intensity, and time. Fitness walking is very effective in increasing or maintaining cardiorespiratory fitness.

Aerobics. Many churches, schools, fitness centers, and community recreational programs now offer aerobics classes. Both men and women enjoy these calisthenics and stretching routines accompanied by music. The aerobic exercises should be either moderate- or low-impact and taught by certified instructors. High-impact aerobics (HIA) results in numerous injuries to its participants and should be avoided. Moderate-impact aerobics (MIA) successfully combines some high and moderate moves and has the same appeal as high-impact aerobics. Low-impact aerobics (LIA) is very good for beginning, overweight, or older individuals. Step aerobics uses low benches to increase the intensity level. Water aerobics is also popular, as well as beneficial in maintaining and improving your fitness. If properly performed, aerobics will be fun and will help you to improve your fitness level.

Games.   Game-type activities are very enjoyable and maintain or improve your cardiorespiratory fitness level if frequency, intensity, and time are sufficient to provide a training stimulus. However, when opponents are not of equal ability, it is sometimes difficult for each participant to receive a training stimulus. Remember, if you use recreational games for a training program, the training stimulus must be sufficient with respect to frequency, intensity, and time.

Recreational games used for cardiorespiratory training also have some disadvantages. These types of activities often require you to make quick starts, stops, and turns or cuts. These quick moves provide greater chance of injury to the joints, tendons, and muscles. A good warm-up is very important before recreational games.

Parcourse.   Many parks, recreational centers, and even housing developments are now building parcourses. A parcourse consists of several exercise stations located along a jogging trail. Parcourses are excellent for improving both cardiorespiratory fitness and muscular endurance. More information concerning parcourses is available in Chapter 5.

INTERVAL TRAINING

Slow, continuous activity is used to build an aerobic base in a cardiorespiratory training program. Such activity permits physiological changes in the body to occur with little chance of injury. In addition, low-intensity, long-duration exercise produces less soreness in the working muscles than high-intensity, short-duration exercise.

As your fitness level improves, the desire for competition may increase. The focus of the training program then shifts from maintaining cardiorespiratory fitness to improving performance. The training principles discussed in Chapter 2 now come into play. In order to increase your performance, you must train at a higher level. A popular method of training to increase your speed is called **interval training.** The following factors are controlled in interval training: distance of the interval, time of the interval, type of recovery between intervals, amount of recovery between intervals, and the number of intervals. For example, interval training in running might involve running a distance of 400 meters in 59 seconds. The recovery period may be a 45-second walk. The runner repeats this sequence until completing 10 intervals.

Adjust your interval training to meet your needs. Most athletes use interval training twice a week. Remember to alternate hard and easy workout days. Interval training is vital when competing in speed and endurance events.

Upon cessation of exercise the heart rate falls, permitting more time for blood to fill the heart. This results in a strong expansion stimulus exerted on the heart, which in turn increases stroke volume. Since interval training consists of repeated periods of intense activity interspersed with recovery periods, the repeated attainment of peak stroke volumes stimulates the oxygen transport system more than standard training methods, in which the only recovery period may occur at the end of the workout. Therefore, most experts agree that interval training best improves stroke volume.

CORONARY DISEASE

A deterioration of cardiorespiratory fitness leads to **C**oronary **D**isease (CD). CD is defined as a disease resulting from changes in the arteries supplying the heart and a subsequent interference with blood flow. It is the greatest cause of death from disease in the United States today. The results of severe, untreated coronary disease include heart attacks and strokes. The likelihood of developing CD is increased by the presence of one or more of the risk factors listed below. Each of these risk factors can add significantly to the chance of suffering a heart attack or stroke. When several risk factors are combined, the probability of developing CD becomes even greater.

RISK FACTORS OF CORONARY DISEASE

The American College of Sports Medicine recognizes increased cholesterol levels, cigarette smoking, and hypertension as the three most influential risk factors for coronary disease. Other factors include physical inactivity, improper diet, obesity, personality and stress, age, genetic factors, gender, and race.

Cholesterol Levels. Many factors contribute to CD; however, your cholesterol levels appear to be the greatest risk factor. The risk of developing CD is an exponential function of the total plasma cholesterol. Your cholesterol level should generally be below 200 mg/dl. The average cholesterol level of a man who has a heart attack is 244 mg/dl. Although total cholesterol is a strong indicator of possible coronary disease, low-density lipoprotein (LDL) cholesterol is a better indicator, and high-density lipoprotein (HDL) cholesterol, as a negative factor, is yet a better indicator.

Increased levels of HDL appear to offer a protective effect against CD for two reasons. First, HDL helps prevent plaque from developing on the walls of blood vessels. Second, HDL appears to be capable of picking up excess fats from the blood and transporting them to the liver for elimination.

The best indicator for determining your risk factor for CD appears to be *your ratio of total cholesterol to high density cholesterol (CHL:HDL).* In a recent study, 90 percent of the individuals whose ratio of CHL:HDL exceeded 6 were found to have significant CD. However, 90 percent of the individuals whose ratio was lower than 3.8 had no significant CD. Generally, you should be treated to lower your CHL:HDL ratio if it exceeds 4.5. The treatment normally includes a change in diet and an increase in physical activity. Sometimes medication is prescribed if you are unable to comply with a more vigorous lifestyle and a prudent diet.

The importance of the ratio of total cholesterol to high-density cholesterol (CHL:HDL) is demonstrated by the following example. If your total cholesterol is 180 mg/dl, you may feel that all is well because it is below 200 mg/dl. However, if your HDL is only 30 mg/dl, then the ratio of CHL:HDL is 6.0 and you would be considered to have a high risk for CD even though your total CHL is not that high.

Smoking. Smoking, especially cigarette smoking, is harmful to your health. Cigarette smokers run about one and one-half times the risk of CD of those who do not smoke. Stopping smoking significantly decreases the risk of developing heart disease. In addition to CD, smoking is linked to cancer, bronchitis, and emphysema. Furthermore, smoking by pregnant women results in an increased risk of premature births, spontaneous abortions, and stillbirths.

Hypertension. Hypertension is chronically elevated blood pressure. Along with bad cholesterol (high LDL or low HDL) levels and smoking, hypertension is one of the greatest risk factors for coronary heart disease. If your blood pressure and cholesterol levels are normal and you do not smoke, your chance of having a heart attack before the age of 65 is less than one in 20. If you have one of these risk factors, your risk doubles. If you have two of these risk factors, your chances are one in two.

Exercise and Diet. Physical inactivity and an improper diet also contribute to heart disease. Physical activity has a positive effect on your cholesterol levels and blood pressure. Studies conducted over a 26-year period involving approximately 3,000 subjects show that vigorous exercise produces beneficial changes in blood lipids and lipoproteins that lower the CHL:HDL ratio. Additionally, exercise tends to lower the blood pressure in individuals suffering from mild or moderate hypertension.

Diet can also affect both cholesterol levels and blood pressure. Your CHL:HDL ratio can be lowered by eating foods low in saturated (animal) fats and by emphasizing vegetables, cereals, lean meats such as fish and fowl, and skim milk in your diet. Generally, you can lower your blood pressure by decreasing your ingestion of salt to five grams per day. Chapter 6 provides more information on diet.

Obesity. Many experts list obesity as a risk factor of CD since obese people often suffer from high blood pressure, which places unnecessary strain on the heart and blood vessels. Most individuals are able to control their weight through diet and vigorous exercise. Chapter 7 provides more information on body composition and weight control.

Personality and Stress. Inability to cope with emotional stress can also contribute to CD. The drive for peer acceptance and success in contemporary society can force an individual to live and work continually faster, leading to disorders such as gastric ulcers, high blood pressure, and migraine headaches. These physical ills are often indicators of excessive mental stress and a corresponding inability to cope with it. Some studies on personality suggest that certain individuals with overly aggressive tendencies and incessant drives to achieve more in less time are constantly under severe mental stress and tension and are likely candidates for CD. Their less-aggressive counterparts are less likely to experience stress-related CD. Chapter 8 provides more information on stress management.

Age. The incidence of CD increases with age. Much of this increase results from physiological deterioration attributable to sedentary living rather than to aging itself. Longitudinal studies show that much of the decline in physical fitness accompanying age can be retarded through regular physical activity.

Genetic Factors. Heredity plays an important role in the development of CD, especially where there is a family history of high blood pressure, high blood-fat levels, or diabetes. Some speculation exists, however, that such relationships may be as much environmental as genetic in nature; that lifestyles and health habits of offspring often parallel those of their parents or other adult role models. For example, hypertensive parents often foster hypertensive children; and obese, inactive parents often have obese, inactive children.

Gender and Race.   Marked differences exist in the incidence of CD with respect to gender and race. Between the ages of 35 and 44, the death rate of white American males is six times greater than that of white American females. After menopause, the incidence of CD for white females nearly approximates that of white males of comparable age. Medical experts believe that the female's diminished hormone production at menopause is responsible for the increased coronary disease rate.

In the case of race, black Americans appear to be more susceptible to CD than white Americans. This is true for both males and females.

Although CD remains one of the leading causes of death in the United States, recent health statistics indicate an encouraging downward trend in the CD death rate. Most experts believe this turnabout is the result of Americans changing their lifestyles to include a prudent diet, more exercise, less smoking, and better control of high blood pressure.

SUPPLEMENTARY READINGS

American Red Cross. *Swimming and Diving.* St. Louis, MO: Mosby–Year Book, 1992.

Brown, A. M., and D. W. Stubbs. *Medical Physiology.* New York: John Wiley & Sons, 1983.

Brown, H. Larry. *Swim Conditioning.* Dubuque, IA: Kendall/Hunt, 1990.

Castelli, W. P. "Epidemiology of Coronary Heart Disease: The Framingham Study." *The American Journal of Medical Sciences,* Vol. 20, 1983.

Chastain, S. M. *Aerobics: A Guide for Participants.* 2d ed. Dubuque, IA: Kendall/Hunt, 1993.

Cooper, K. "If You are Running More Than 3 Miles, 5 Times a Week. . . ." *Inside Aerobics,* 1984.

Counsilman, James E., and Brian E. Counsilman. *The New Science of Swimming.* Englewood Cliffs, NJ: Prentice Hall, 1994.

Draper, D. O., and G. L. Jones. "The 1.5-Mile Run Revisited—An Update in Women's Times." *Journal of Physical Education, Recreation and Dance,* Vol. 61, No. 7, pp. 78–80, September 1990.

Friedman, M., and R. H. Rosenman. *Type A Behavior and Your Heart.* New York: Knopf, 1974.

Hoeger, W. W. K. *Fitness and Wellness.* 2d ed. Englewood, CO: Morton Publishing, 1993.

Hollman, W., et al. "The Importance of Sport and Physical Training in Preventive Cardiology." *The Journal of Sports Medicine and Physical Fitness,* Vol. 20, No. 1, March 1980.

Kusinitz, I., and M. Fine. *Your Guide to Getting Fit.* 2d ed. Mountain View, CA: Mayfield Publishing, 1991.

Maglischo, E. W. *Swimming Even Faster: A Comprehensive Guide to the Science of Swimming.* 2d ed. Mountain View, CA: Mayfield Publishing, 1993.

Marley, W. P. *Health and Physical Fitness.* Dubuque, IA: Wm. C. Brown, 1988.

Nieman, D. C. *Fitness and Your Health.* Palo Alto, CA: Bull Publishing, 1993.

Rosato, F. *Jogging for Health and Fitness.* Englewood, CO: Morton Publishing, 1988.

Schwartz, C. C., et al. "Preferential Utilization of Free Cholesterol from High-Density Lipoproteins for Biliary Cholesterol Secretion in Man." *Science,* Vol. 200, pp. 62–64, April 7, 1978.

Segrest, J. P., et al. "Coronary Heart Disease Risk: Assessment by Plasma Lipoprotein Profiles." *The Alabama Journal of Medical Sciences,* Vol. 20, 1983.

Seiger, L. H. and J. Hesson. *Walking for Fitness.* 2d ed. Madison, WI: Brown & Benchmark, 1994.

Tidus, P. M., and C. P. Ianuzzo. "Effects of Intensity and Duration of Muscular Exercise on Delayed Soreness and Serum Enzyme Activities." *Medicine and Science in Sports and Exercise,* Vol. 15, No. 6, 1983.

Vu Tran, C., et al. "The Effect of Exercise on Blood Lipids and Lipoproteins: A Meta-Analysis of Studies." *Medicine and Science in Sports and Exercise,* Vol. 15, No. 5, 1983.

Zampogna, A., et al. "Relationship Between Lipids and Occlusive Artery Disease." *Archives of Internal Medicine,* Vol. 140, p. 1067, 1980.

CHAPTER 4 REVIEW QUESTIONS

1. Which component of fitness do most physical fitness experts consider to be the most important?

2. What are *aerobic* activities?

3. What is recommended in regard to frequency, intensity, and time when training for cardiorespiratory fitness?
   a. frequency:

   b. intensity:

   c. time:

4. Describe how you should warm up.

5. How can you avoid overtraining?

6. Describe some symptoms that should warn you to discontinue your workout.

7. Describe how you should cool down.

8. What is the most accurate way to assess cardiorespiratory fitness?

9. Describe how you should monitor your heart rate.

10. List at least four benefits you can expect from a cardiorespiratory training program.

11. What are some advantages and disadvantages of the following cardiorespiratory training activities?

   a. jogging
      advantages:

      disadvantages:

   b. cycling
      advantages:

      disadvantages:

   c. swimming
      advantages:

      disadvantages:

   d. fitness walking
      advantages:

      disadvantages:

   e. aerobics
      advantages:

      disadvantages:

f. games

advantages:

disadvantages:

12. What is a parcourse?

13. What is interval training?

14. List nine factors that contribute to coronary disease.
a.

b.

c.

d.

e.

f.

g.

h.

i.

15. What appears to be the best indicator for determining your risk of coronary heart disease?

16. How can you improve your cholesterol levels?

17. List at least three hazards of smoking.

18. What is hypertension?

19. How do diet and exercise affect your risk of coronary disease?

20. How are most individuals able to control their weight?

21. What is the correlation between stress and your risk of coronary disease?

22. What is the correlation between age and your risk of coronary disease?

23. What role does heredity play in the development of coronary disease?

24. How do race and gender affect your risk of coronary disease?

5

Muscular Strength and Endurance

This chapter deals with the development of muscular strength and endurance. Strength is the maximum force that a muscle or muscle group can exert against resistance during a single effort. Endurance is the ability of a muscle or muscle group to exert force for an extended period of time. Benefits from a strength-and-endurance training program include increased muscle mass and strength, improved posture and vitality, and positive self-image. Furthermore, research in weight control indicates that a decline in metabolism, found in individuals as they age, primarily results from a decrease in muscle mass. Therefore, continuing a strength-and-endurance training program will aid in the battle against creeping obesity, which is discussed in Chapter 7.

TYPES OF MUSCULAR CONTRACTION

The normal response of a muscle fiber to a training stimulus is the development of force directed longitudinally. The amount of force developed by the muscle compared to the opposing force determines the type of muscular contraction.

Concentric Contraction. If the force developed by the muscle is greater than the opposing force, the muscle shortens and thus performs work. This type of contraction, in which the muscle shortens, is called a concentric contraction.

Eccentric Contraction. If the force developed by the muscle is less than the opposing force, the muscle lengthens. This type of contraction is referred to as an eccentric contraction.

Isometric Contraction. If the force developed by the muscle balances the opposing force, the muscle remains at a constant length. This type of contraction is called an isometric contraction.

Examples of concentric, eccentric, and isometric contraction occur when performing pull-ups to exhaustion. As you pull your body to the bar, you have concentric contraction of the biceps and latissimus dorsi muscle groups. As you lower your body away from the bar, eccentric contraction occurs. Isometric contraction occurs when you reach the point at which you are attempting to raise your body to the bar but are unable to move upward.

SKELETAL MOVEMENT AND MUSCLE ACTIONS

Voluntary movement of your skeletal system is brought about by the shortening of skeletal muscles. There are over 400 skeletal muscles in your body. These muscles are attached to the bones by tendons. In order for skeletal movement to occur, it is necessary that a muscle be attached to at least two different bones. Normally, each muscle acting upon a joint is matched by another muscle called an antagonist, which has an opposite action. For example, the biceps brachii (an elbow flexor) and the triceps brachii (an elbow extensor) are antagonists at the elbow. Most movements require the combined action of a number of muscles. Those muscles that act directly to bring about a desired movement are called **prime movers.** Supporting muscles that hold the part of the body being acted upon in the appropriate position are called **fixation** muscles. The drawing on page 61 illustrates the major muscle groups of the body.

GENETIC FACTORS

It is important to realize that genetic factors affect physical performance. These factors include the number of muscle fibers in a muscle group, the type of muscle fiber that is predominant in the muscle group, and the structure of the muscle fibers in the muscle group.

Number of Muscle Fibers.   Each muscle of the body consists of groups of muscle bundles that join into a tendon at each end. These bundles in turn consist of thousands of muscle fibers or cells. In humans, the number of muscle fibers in a muscle group is established after the embryo has reached the age of four to five months. However, you can alter the thickness of the fiber with training.

Types of Muscle Fibers.   There are two main types of fibers in the skeletal muscle: fast-twitch and slow-twitch. The muscles of the body consist of a combination of these two major fiber types. The proportion of fast-twitch fibers ranges from about 5 to 90 percent of the total. The higher the proportion of fast-twitch fibers, the faster the whole muscle contracts.

Muscles having predominantly slow-twitch fibers are used for prolonged performance of work. These slow-twitch fibers are generally smaller, are surrounded by more blood capillaries, and have more mitochondria (which are responsible for the conversion of food to useful energy) than the fast-twitch fibers do. The mitochondria are sometimes called the **powerhouse** of the muscle cell due to the fact that adenosine triphosphate (ATP)—the energy source required for muscular activity—is formed there. Slow-twitch fibers also have a large amount of myoglobin, which gives a red tint to the fiber. Due to this red tint, slow-twitch fibers are sometimes referred to as red fibers and fast-twitch as white fibers. Myoglobin is a substance similar to the hemoglobin in red blood cells and can combine with and store oxygen inside the muscle cell until needed by the mitochondria.

Fast-twitch fibers normally allow a very rapid release and subsequent absorption of calcium ions so that the contraction occurs quickly. Individuals with predominantly fast-twitch fibers are normally better suited for speed activities, while individuals with predominantly slow-twitch fibers are better suited for endurance activities.

Structure of Muscle Fibers.   There are two major fiber structures in your skeletal muscle: **fusiform** and **pennate.** The fusiform muscle fibers run longitudinally and relatively parallel to the muscle's long axis. A single fiber does not run the entire length of the muscle, but the many fibers that make up the muscle are aligned as a group with the muscle's long axis. The pennate muscle fibers run obliquely to the muscle's longitudinal axis but have tendons that run parallel with the muscle's long axis.

The fusiform, or longitudinal, fibers are longer and can shorten a greater effective distance than the pennate, or oblique, fibers; therefore, the fusiform can pull the bones through a greater range of motion. However, there are fewer fusiform fibers per unit of area than there are pennate or oblique fibers. Thus, the fusiform fibers can pull the bones through greater range of motion, but the pennate fibers are capable of generating more force. The proportion of fusiform to pennate fibers in the muscle determines the range of motion and the amount of force that the muscle is capable of producing.

These are just a few of the genetic factors affecting human performance. Heredity definitely plays an important role and establishes the upper limit in human performance. However, few individuals ever reach the state of training in which they begin to approach their potential.

GENDER

The sex hormone level affects the capacity for muscular size development. The popular myth that exercise, especially resistance exercise, tends to masculinize the physical appearance of women has no basis for most women. The muscle fibers of both sexes are similar, both histochemically and distributionally. However, females have a smaller cross-sectional area in all fiber types than males. Higher levels of androgens in males account for much of the muscle hypertrophy and strength differences between the sexes. Androgens are hormones that develop and maintain masculine characteristics. Since women have lower levels of androgens, it is very unlikely that they will obtain the muscle size and strength of men. Women and older men, with lower levels of androgens, apparently gain strength by improving their ability to recruit additional motor units rather than by significantly altering the contractile structure of the muscles.

PROGRESSIVE-RESISTANCE EXERCISE

In order for a muscle cell to increase in size and strength, you must increase its workload beyond what it normally experiences. Muscles adapt to the workload you place upon them. When this adaptation takes place, you must place a greater workload on the muscle in order to achieve further gains. Progressively increasing the stress (workload) placed on the muscle as adaptation takes place is referred to as **progressive-resistance** exercise (PRE). The three most common forms of progressive-resistance exercise are isotonic, isometric, and isokinetic.

Isotonic Training.   Isotonic training, commonly called weight training, is characterized by the exertion of force on movable objects such as barbells, dumbbells, and pulley weights. It is used extensively in athletic conditioning to develop muscular power or explosive strength, which is a maximal strength output over a very short period of time. In isotonic training a series of exercises selected to involve all the major muscles of the body are performed against varying amounts of resistance. One completion of the exercise is called a **repetition,** and a series of these repetitions, performed consecutively, is called an exercise **set.**

Isometric Training.   Isometric training involves nonmoving or static muscle contractions performed against immovable objects such as a wall or a door frame, or against one's own opposing (antagonistic) muscles. Researchers have found that static contraction of muscles at two-thirds of maximum effort for six seconds can increase strength. Such strength increases, however, are related directly to the specific joint angle at which the isometric contraction occurs. For example, if you repeatedly performed isometric arm contractions with the elbow bent at 90 degrees, maximum strength gains will be at that angle but gains will be less at other angles through the range of motion.

Isometric exercises have some advantages over other forms of resistance exercises: they require little space and no special equipment, and isometrics can be performed almost anywhere. Physical therapy programs often employ isometrics or isotonics to rehabilitate muscles weakened by injury or disease.

Isokinetic Training.   A muscular contraction is isokinetic when the speed of the contraction is kept constant against a variable resistance. Isokinetic training makes use of a specialized apparatus, such as the Syber machine, that provides variable resistance directly proportional to the amount of muscular force being applied by the exerciser and controls and holds the speed of movement constant during the exercise. This permits a muscle or group of muscles to encounter maximum resistance throughout a complete range of motion. This accommodating resistance allows more muscular work to be performed and reduces the likelihood of muscle strain, which can occur when attempting to overcome a **sticking point** during isotonic training or when trying to move an immovable object in isometric training. The Nautilus system, although it provides maximum resistance throughout the range of motion, is not a true isokinetic process because it allows for unrestricted speed of movement. It is, however, an effective and popular means of developing strength.

Once in a weight training program, you can expect some improvement in strength in four to six weeks. Two factors strongly influence the rate and extent of improvement: your starting level of fitness and the intensity and regularity of your workouts. Genetic factors affecting the quality of muscle tissue and your personal drive or motivation also control strength development.

Most, though not all, studies comparing the various forms of resistance exercise conclude that all three methods described can produce significant strength gains in relatively short periods of time. Recent research seems to indicate that isokinetic resistance training is superior to the other methods for strength gains.

MUSCULAR STRENGTH/ENDURANCE TRAINING GUIDELINES

Warm-Up.   A warm-up should precede all training activities. It consists of three phases: cardiorespiratory, flexibility, and muscular endurance. First perform a cardiorespiratory activity such as rope skipping or running in place at a moderate rate to elevate the heart rate and body temperature. Then use flexibility exercises to prevent musculoskeletal injuries. Next perform submaximal muscular-endurance activities to prepare the working muscles for the greater stress that will follow in the workout. You should then perform several repetitions of your workout exercises with very light resistance for the final phase of the warm-up.

Cool-Down. The cool-down following most progressive-resistance training programs consists mainly of stretching exercises to help improve the flexibility of the joints. In general, progressive-resistance training programs place little demand on the cardiorespiratory system; therefore, little time is needed to allow the heart and lungs to recover. This is not the case for circuit training, which is discussed later in this chapter. The cool-down after circuit training requires time for the cardiorespiratory system to recover in addition to the flexibility phase.

Breathing. In progressive-resistance exercise there is a tendency to hold your breath as the fixation muscles attempt to provide a base from which the prime movers can apply leverage. When the breath is held, the pressure within the thoracic cavity increases as the chest compresses from the actions of the working muscles. This can cause a sudden and dramatic rise in blood pressure, which reduces the return of blood to the heart. A drop in blood pressure, which may cause dizziness or fainting, follows. This series of events is referred to as the **Valsalva phenomenon** and can be easily prevented by not holding your breath during exercise. The Valsalva phenomenon is particularly dangerous if you have high blood pressure. The rule to follow regarding breathing during progressive-resistance exercise is to *inhale as the chest is expanding and exhale as the chest compresses.* This means that in most pushing exercises, such as the bench press, you would exhale during exertion and inhale during recovery. In most pulling exercises, such as a pull-up, you should inhale on exertion and exhale on recovery.

Lifting Safety. Always use proper form when lifting objects. When lifting an object such as a barbell from the floor, begin with your feet comfortably spread and toes pointed ahead. Lower your hips to a squat position by bending the knees. Keep your head up and back straight. Begin the lifting motion with your legs, not your back.

Exercises that start with a barbell at the chest or shoulders employ a preliminary movement in which the barbell is raised from the floor to the chest or shoulders in one uninterrupted movement known as a **clean**. The starting position for the clean is the squat position described above. The movement involves a forceful straightening of your legs, followed by an upward pull of the bar with your arms. After you overcome the force of inertia and the barbell is rising, bend your knees slightly and take a small step forward to help in bringing the barbell to your chest; then straighten your legs.

When lifting heavy barbells in the squat, bench press, or overhead lifts, always have one or more spotters standing by to assist in removing the weight should you lose control. When using adjustable barbells and dumbbells, always check to make sure that collars holding the weight plates in place are properly fastened to prevent them from sliding off the bar. With machines, check cables for premature wearing and make sure that the weight-adjusting pin is securely in place.

Form. Exercises should be completed using good form in order to avoid injury.

To maximize work output, perform weight training exercises slowly and deliberately. During the **concentric** phase of an exercise, when working muscles are contracting (the *up* movement of the barbell), be careful not to swing or jerk the barbell upward. Likewise, during the **eccentric** phase, when working muscles are stretching (the *down* movement of the barbell), strive to maintain steady tension on the working muscles by lowering the weight slowly and not allowing the force of gravity to do the work.

The term **muscle-boundness** implies decreased flexibility, quickness, and coordination. The notion that progressive-resistance training causes this condition is unfounded. Weight trainers who have achieved international recognition for their muscular development or for competitive weight lifting ability have been found to possess above-average joint flexibility and speed of movement. However, a decrease in joint mobility will result if you consistently fail to perform weight training exercises through the full range of motion, do not use flexibility exercises, and fail to strengthen the antagonist muscle groups. The one exception to performing exercises through their full range of motion is the squat exercise. Because of the structure of the knee joint, ligament injury can occur to this joint in the deep squat (completely flexed) position.

Selection and Sequence of Exercises.   Total-body development is necessary to ensure symmetrical muscular development and prevent loss of joint mobility. Select exercises that will strengthen all of the major muscle groups. Also, avoid the pitfall of constantly using the same exercises in your workout. You will find that you can increase overall strength of each muscle group by slightly varying some of the exercises in your workout program periodically. This recruits additional muscle fibers in the muscle group and thus results in greater overall development.

The sequence for exercising should progress from large- to small-muscle groups. Those exercises that develop the large-muscle groups of the body—squats, cleans, and presses—should form the basis of your program. The amount of time you have for training will influence the exercises you choose for your workout. If your time is limited, your workout should comprise exercises that develop large-muscle groups. These exercises will usually develop smaller-muscle groups in addition to the large muscles. For example, the bench press develops the anterior deltoids and triceps in addition to the large pectoral muscles. Add exercises that develop the smaller-muscle groups as time permits. Appendix B provides a Muscular Strength/Endurance Training Record log for you to record your progressive-resistance exercise workouts.

Frequency, Intensity, and Time.   The rate of improvement in muscular strength and endurance is dependent upon the frequency, intensity, and time of training. Generally, training sessions should be on alternate days, three times per week.

When beginning a program, you should be conservative regarding the starting resistance for each exercise. Initially, choose a resistance that you are sure you can easily perform for 10 to 15 repetitions. After you develop proper form, then increase the resistance as desired.

A resistance that represents 60 to 80 percent of a muscle's maximal strength is sufficient to produce increases in strength. Generally, such a workload permits the completion of seven to ten repetitions. If you are just beginning a program, you should perform all exercises with workloads that permit the performance of a single set of seven to ten repetitions. When skill and strength improvement permit you to perform correctly more than ten repetitions under maximal (overload) conditions, increase the resistance five to ten pounds for succeeding workouts.

The amount of time you should spend training depends upon your goals and the demands on your time of other factors in your life. If other demands limit your time, you should use exercises that incorporate large muscles. If time is not a factor, you should supplement your large-muscle-group exercises with exercises that develop individual muscles. The amount of time you rest between sets depends upon your goals. The rest between sets normally varies from 30 seconds when using light resistance for improving muscular endurance to four or five minutes when using heavy resistance for improving strength. Many individuals who lift for general fitness use a rest period of one to two minutes.

DESIGNING YOUR MUSCULAR STRENGTH/ENDURANCE PROGRAM

The amount of success you experience in your muscular strength/endurance program will be determined in large part by your commitment and how you design your program.

Consider the following factors when designing your program: goals, simplicity, completeness, progression, and variety.

Goals.   Before attempting to set goals, you should thoroughly understand the training principles discussed in Chapter 2, as well as the selection and sequence of exercises and training guidelines (regarding frequency, intensity, and time) discussed in this chapter. Your goals must be realistic. Setting easily attainable short-range goals will help you reach your long-range goals. Write down your goals and then keep a log of workouts to help monitor your progress. There is a Fitness Evaluation Record in Appendix B for you to record your starting values for several muscular strength and endurance exercises.

Simplicity and Completeness.   Your core program should consist of the fewest number of exercises needed to reach your goals. Your workout should include at least one exercise that will work each of the major muscle groups in the body. If time permits, add exercises that work smaller groups. Remember to progress from large- to small-muscle groups.

Progression and Variety.   You must follow the training guidelines with respect to frequency, intensity, and time in order to stress the muscles for strength or endurance. Also, remember to increase the intensity as your body adapts. Your workouts should be cyclic in nature. Vary the intensity of the workouts. Don't make every workout the same. Periodically, substitute other exercises to develop the same large-muscle groups. This will recruit different fibers of the same large-muscle group and will result in greater strength gains. Using a mix of exercise modes—for example, free weights, machines, and calisthenics—will add variety to your program.

WEIGHT TRAINING

Weight training is the most popular form of progressive-resistance training. The variety of systems used in weight training can be geared to your specific needs, priorities, and preferences.

Progressive.   This is the recommended system for individuals beginning a training program. Keep the number of repetitions constant but increase the resistance as you make gains in strength.

Light and Heavy.   In this system, you normally perform three to five sets. Perform the first set against the maximum resistance that allows five to eight repetitions. On each succeeding set, increase resistance, which will cause the number of repetitions to decrease. Continue until you can perform only one repetition.

Pyramid.   This is similar to the light-and-heavy system except that the procedure is reversed after reaching the one-repetition plateau, and you work back down the resistance scale.

Superset.   A superset consists of a set for one muscle group immediately followed by a set for its antagonist. An example is alternating a set of upright curls for the biceps and a set of tricep presses for the triceps. A multiple superset involves simply repeating the paired exercises for two or more exercise sets.

Multiple Sets.   In this system you attempt to perform a series of sets using the same resistance and the same number of repetitions. Normally, the number of repetitions decreases with each succeeding set due to fatigue.

Blitz. If you find that you do not have enough time to train as long as you desire each training session, you can divide your workout training period into smaller units of time but train more days each week. For example, you can divide a three-hour workout session of thirty or more exercises into three different and distinct workouts of ten exercises each. Monday's workout may consist of arm and shoulder exercises, Tuesday's workout may consist of chest and back exercises, and Wednesday's workout may consist of leg and abdominal exercises. The progression would be repeated on Thursday, Friday, and Saturday, with Sunday being a rest day. Such a program permits the serious weight trainer to lift six days per week but still provides adequate rest for the muscles to recover from the intense workouts.

GETTING STARTED WITH WEIGHT TRAINING

Many students are hesitant to begin a training program for a number of reasons. Two of the most commonly cited are not knowing where to begin and feeling intimidated in the weight room by those more muscular and fit. The first concern is easily overcome by establishing personal goals and developing a training program that will allow you to meet these goals. Addressing the second concern requires the self-confidence to ignore the fitness level of others and to progress at your own pace.

In addition to your personal goals regarding the development of muscular strength and endurance, a beginning weight training program should

1. exercise all the major muscle groups of the body
2. develop the body symmetrically (reinforces #1)
3. focus on multijoint exercises that work large-muscle groups
4. consist of around 10 exercises with alternate exercises to provide variation

Following is a basic program that will get you started and, with occasional modification, continue to aid you in developing total-body muscular strength and endurance. Detailed information concerning the performance of these exercises is provided later in the chapter. You may use variations of the exercises listed. It is neither necessary nor advisable for the beginner to perform all the variations during a single workout. Rather, these exercises provide variety in your workout to ensure total development and to help avoid boredom.

BEGINNING MUSCULAR STRENGTH AND ENDURANCE TRAINING PROGRAM

EXERCISE	BODY AREAS EXERCISED
1. Bench press (Figures 5.1, 5.2)	Chest, shoulders, back upper arms
2. Overhead press (Figures 5.3, 5.4)	Shoulders, upper back, back upper arms
3. Upright row (Figures 5.9, 5.10)	Upper back, shoulders, front upper arms
4. Lat pulldown (Figures 5.5, 5.6)	Back, front upper arms
5. Curl-ups (Figure 5.35)	Abdominals
6. Back extensions (Figures 5.21, 5.22)	Back
7. Half-squat (Figures 5.25, 5.26)	Buttocks, front upper legs, back upper legs, lower back
8. Leg extensions (Figures 5.15, 5.16)	Front upper legs
9. Leg curls (Figures 5.17, 5.18)	Buttocks, back upper legs
10. Heel raise (Figures 5.19, 5.20)	Back lower legs
11. Upright curl (Figures 5.13, 5.14)	Front upper arms
12. Tricep extensions (Figures 5.11, 5.12)	Back upper arms

MAJOR MUSCLE GROUPS OF THE BODY

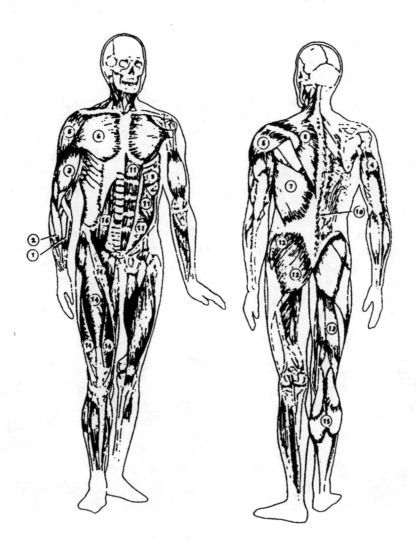

1. Forearm flexors
2. Brachioradialis
3. Biceps
4. Triceps
5. Deltoid
6. Pectoral muscles
7. Latissimus dorsi
8. Trapezius
9. Serratus anterior
10. Erector spinae (spinal extensors)
11. Abdominal muscles
    a. Internal and external obliques
    b. Rectus abdominis
    c. Transversalis
12. Gluteal muscles
13. Hamstrings
14. Quadriceps muscles
15. Gastrocnemius, soleus muscles
16. Iliopsoas (under abdominal muscles)

Adapted from *Muscle Action Chart Number 10* by V. F. Krumdick and Cramer Products, Inc.

MUSCULAR STRENGTH/ENDURANCE TRAINING EXERCISES

Bench Press

Major muscle groups: Pectorals (chest), deltoids (shoulders), and triceps (back upper arms).

Starting position (Figure 5.1): Lie in the supine position (face up) on the bench with your feet flat on the floor. Hold the barbell with a pronated grip (palms facing away), with your hands slightly wider than shoulder-width apart and your arms fully extended above your chest.

Movement (Figure 5.2): Slowly lower the barbell until it touches your chest. Raise the barbell to full extension of your arms to complete one repetition. Your head, shoulders, and buttocks should remain in contact with the bench throughout the entire exercise. Keep your feet flat on the floor.

Precaution: Use spotters. Avoid bouncing the bar off your chest. **Do not arch your back off the bench, as this results in hyperextension of the lower back.** Some individuals prefer to place their feet on the bench instead of the floor to avoid hyperextension of the lower back. Be extra careful when doing this because your base of support is much smaller when your feet are on the bench. With your feet on the bench, you may experience problems balancing the barbell as you go through the movement.

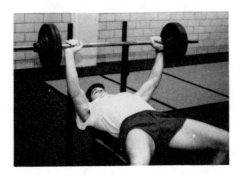 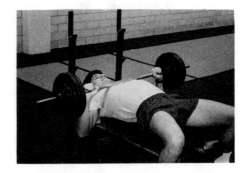

Figure 5.1   **Figure 5.2**

Seated Overhead Press

Major muscle groups: Deltoids (shoulders), trapezius (upper back), and triceps (back upper arms).

Starting position (Figure 5.3): Sit with your feet approximately shoulder-width apart. The barbell is in the *clean* position, with the hands using a pronated grip. You may also perform this exercise from a seated position on a bench.

Movement (Figure 5.4): Raise the barbell overhead to a straight-arm position. To recover, slowly lower the barbell to the starting position.

Precaution: Avoid hyperextension or arching of the lower back, since it places undue strain on the lumbar vertebrae. Also, excessive bending of the lower back changes the emphasis of the exercise from the shoulder to the chest.

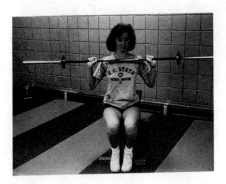

Figure 5.3

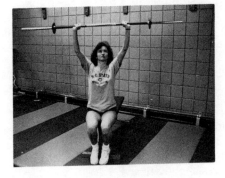

Figure 5.4

Lat Pulls

Major muscle groups: Latissimus dorsi (back), trapezius (upper back), and biceps (front upper arms).

Starting position (Figure 5.5): Using the lat machine, grasp the bar in a pronated grip, with the hands slightly wider than shoulder-width. Kneel or sit, depending on the length of the cable to the pulley. Hold the bar with your arms fully extended overhead.

Movement (Figure 5.6): Pull the bar down behind your head until it touches your shoulders. To recover, allow the bar to be pulled slowly back to the starting position by the force created by the weight stack that is attached to the pulley.

Precaution: Avoid leaning your trunk back as you perform the exercise, since this changes the emphasis of the exercise to the spinal erector muscle in your lower back. Make sure that the weight-stack adjustment pin is secured before beginning the exercise. Avoid contacting the cervical vertebrae as you pull the bar down to your shoulders.

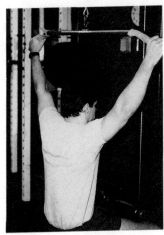

Figure 5.5

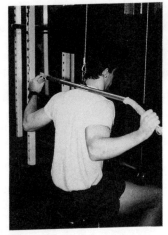

Figure 5.6

Bent Row

Major muscle groups· Rhomboids (upper back), trapezius (upper back), latissimus dorsi (back), and biceps (front upper arms).

Starting position (Figure 5.7): Bend forward at the waist, with your trunk parallel to the floor. Flex your knees, with your feet approximately shoulder-width apart. Using a pronated grip with your hands approximately shoulder-width apart, hold the barbell a couple of inches above the floor with your arms fully extended.

Movement (Figure 5.8): Keeping your torso parallel to the floor and knees slightly flexed, raise the barbell until it touches your chest. To recover, lower the barbell to the starting position.

Precaution: Avoid raising your head and torso. Resting your head on a tabletop reduces some of the strain on your lower back. However, when using a tabletop, keep your neck straight to avoid stress on the cervical vertebrae. Don't lift with straightened knees; keep your knees slightly flexed.

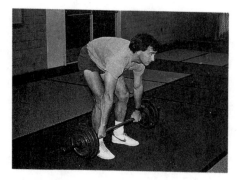

Figure 5.7

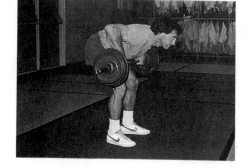

Figure 5.8

Upright Row

Major muscle groups: Trapezius (upper back), deltoids (shoulders), and biceps (front upper arms).

Starting position (Figure 5.9): Stand upright with your feet shoulder-width apart and knees slightly flexed. Hold the barbell with a pronated grip, your arms fully extended and the barbell resting across the front of your thighs. Place your hands approximately six to eight inches apart.

Movement (Figure 5.10): Raise the barbell until the bar is at chin level. Keep your elbows higher than the bar throughout the movement. To recover, slowly lower the barbell to the starting position.

Precaution: Avoid bending backwards. Do not lock or hyperextend the knees during the exercise.

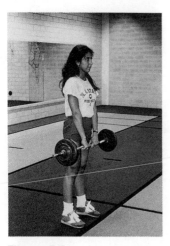

Figure 5.9

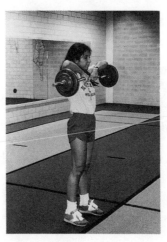

Figure 5.10

Standing Tricep Extension

Major muscle groups: Triceps (back upper arms).

Starting position (Figure 5.11): Stand upright and hold the lat bar with a pronated grip. Position your hands approximately eight inches apart, and bend your elbows approximately 90 degrees.

Movement (Figure 5.12): Keeping your elbows stationary, press the bar down to full extension of the elbows. Slowly return to the starting position. Except for the forearms, your body should remain stationary.

Precaution: Avoid leaning forward at the waist.

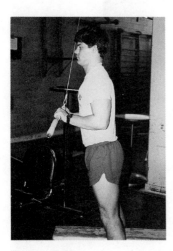

Figure 5.11

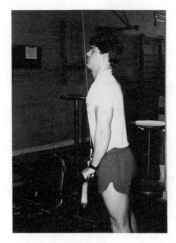

Figure 5.12

Upright Curl

Major muscle groups: Biceps (front upper arms) and brachials (upper arms).

Starting position (Figure 5.13):   Stand with your feet approximately shoulder-width apart, and hold the barbell with a supinated grip in a straight-arm position resting across the front of the thighs. Position your hands approximately shoulder-width apart.

Movement (Figure 5.14):   Raise the barbell forward and upward in an arc toward your chest. Your elbows are the center of the arc and should be held stationary at your sides. To recover, slowly return the barbell through the same plane of movement to the starting position.

Precaution: Avoid bending backwards, and do not arch the back. Keep your body in a straight upright position while doing this exercise. Keep your knees slightly flexed throughout the movement.

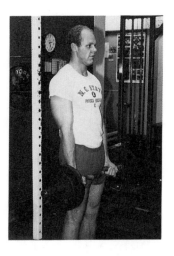

Figure 5.13

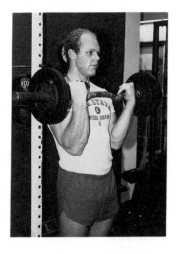

Figure 5.14

Leg Extensions

Major muscle groups: Quadriceps (front upper legs).

Starting position (Figure 5.15):   Sit flat with the padded bar resting just above the ankles on the front of your lower legs.

Movement (Figure 5.16):   Extend the knees almost to the straight-leg position (knees still slightly flexed). To recover, return to a position where the angle of your knees has not quite returned to that of the starting position.

Precaution: Do not hyperextend knees or return to the initial starting position during this exercise, since doing so places harmful pressure on the knee joint.

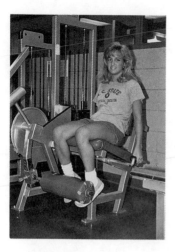

Figure 5.15

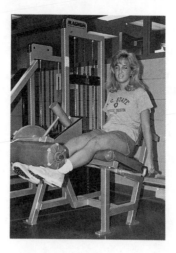

Figure 5.16

Leg Curls

Major muscle groups: Hamstrings (back upper legs).

Starting position (Figure 5.17):   Lie in the prone position (face down) on the bench, with your head down and turned to one side to protect your lower back. The padded bars should rest above the ankles on the back of the lower legs. Hold the handles attached to the bench for support.

Movement (Figure 5.18):   Flex the knees to move the padded bars towards the buttocks as far as possible. To recover, return to the starting position.

Precaution: Perform the exercise in a slow, smooth manner.

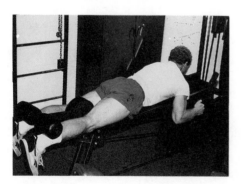

Figure 5.17

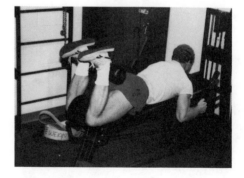

Figure 5.18

Heel Raise

Major muscle groups: Gastrocnemius and soleus (back lower legs).

Starting position: Stand upright with your feet shoulder-width apart. If you are using free weights, the barbell rests across the shoulders, behind the head, and is stabilized by the hands. You can place a block of wood or barbell plate beneath the balls of the feet and toes to maximize the movement. If you are using the Nautilus multiexercise machine (Figure 5.19), secure the waist strap around the hips.

Movement (Figure 5.20): Slowly raise your heels off the floor so that the weight of your body is supported on the toes and balls of your feet. To recover, slowly lower your heels back to the floor.

Precaution: Keep your body in an upright, straight position while doing this exercise. Do *not* hyperextend your knees between lifts.

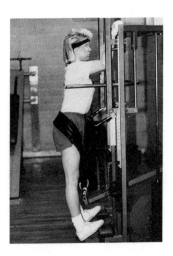

Figure 5.19

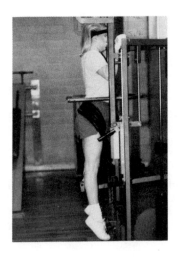

Figure 5.20

Back Extensions

Major muscle groups: Erector spinae (lower back).

Starting position (Figure 5.21): Lie in a prone position on a table or bench, with your feet anchored and your torso hanging down beyond the edge of the bench. Place your hands behind your head.

Movement (Figure 5.22): Lift your head and shoulders until they are slightly higher than parallel to the floor. To recover, slowly lower your torso back to the starting position.

Precaution: Avoid fast, jerking movements and hyperextension of your back, as these movements may cause injury.

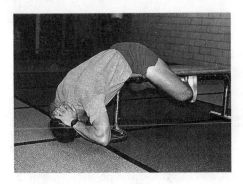

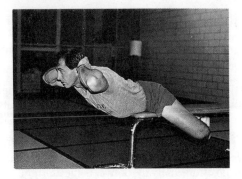

Figure 5.21

Figure 5.22

Shoulder Shrugs

Major muscle groups: Trapezius (upper back) and deltoids (shoulders).

Starting position (Figure 5.23):   Stand upright with your feet shoulder-width apart and knees slightly flexed. Hold the barbell with a pronated grip, the arms fully extended and the barbell resting across the front of your thighs. Space your hands a little wider than shoulder-width apart.

Movement (Figure 5.24):   Raise your shoulders toward your ears in a shrugging motion while holding the barbell at waist level. To recover, slowly lower the barbell to the starting position.

Precaution: Perform the lifting and lowering movements slowly, keeping your arms straight to provide maximum force on the upper trapezius muscles.

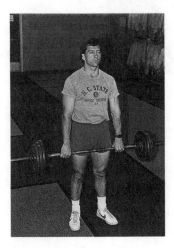

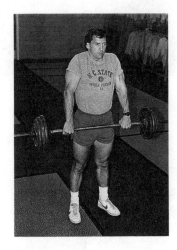

Figure 5.23

Figure 5.24

Half-Squat

Major muscle groups: Gluteus maximus (buttocks), quadriceps (front upper legs), hamstrings (back upper legs), and erector spinae (lower back).

Starting position (Figure 5.25):   Stand upright with your feet approximately shoulder-width apart and toes pointing slightly to the outside. Slightly flex your knees. Rest the barbell on your shoulders behind your head. Hold the barbell in a pronated grip, with your hands slightly wider than shoulder-width apart.

Movement (Figure 5.26):   While keeping the back straight, lower your body to the half-squat position, halfway between the upright position and the full-squat position. Keeping your back straight, return to the starting position.

Precaution: If performed incorrectly, this exercise can cause serious back problems. Avoid leaning forward during the movement as this places undue strain on the lower back. Watching a spot high on a wall as you go through the range of motion often helps keep your back straight. Use light resistance until you have developed good form. Use spotters.

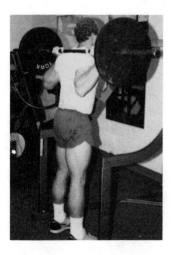

Figure 5.25

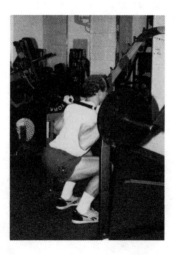

Figure 5.26

Pull-Ups

Major muscle groups: Latissimus dorsi (back) and biceps (front upper arms).

Starting position (Figure 5.27):   Hang from the pull-up bar with your arms fully extended and using a pronated grip (palms facing away from you). The hands should be slightly wider than shoulder-width apart.

Movement (Figure 5.28):   Without kicking, swaying, or jerking, pull your body upward until your chin is above the bar and then slowly lower yourself to the starting position.

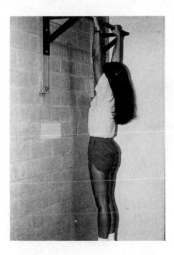

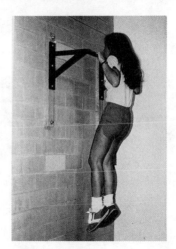

Figure 5.27   Figure 5.28

Push-Ups

Major muscle groups: Pectorals (chest), anterior deltoids (shoulders), and triceps (back upper arms).

Starting position (Figure 5.29):   Lie in a prone position and support your body on your hands and feet with your elbows fully extended. Keep your feet together, hands about shoulder-width apart, back straight, and head down with your eyes looking slightly ahead.

Movement (Figure 5.30):   Keeping your body straight, bend your elbows until your chest touches the floor. Return to the starting position.

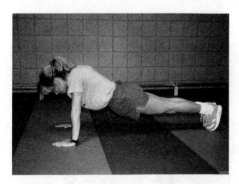

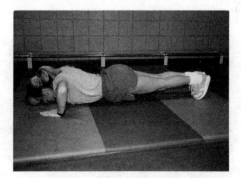

Figure 5.29   Figure 5.30

Modified Push-Ups

Major muscle groups: Pectorals (chest), anterior deltoids (shoulders), and triceps (back upper arms).

Starting position (Figure 5.31):   Lie in a prone position and support your body on your hands and knees, with your elbows fully extended. Keep your knees together, hands about shoulder-width apart, back straight, and head down with your eyes looking slightly ahead.

Movement (Figure 5.32):   Keeping your body straight, bend your elbows until your chest touches the floor. Return to the starting position.

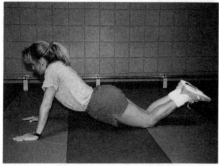

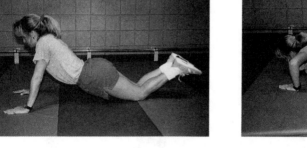

Figure 5.31

Figure 5.32

Bench Dips

Major muscle groups: Triceps (back upper arms) and anterior deltoids (shoulders).

Starting position (Figure 5.33):   Place two stable benches parallel to each other at a distance approximately the length of from your heel to your chest. Rest your heels on one bench and place your hands approximately shoulder-width apart with the elbows extended to support your body, as shown in Figure 5.33.

Movement (Figure 5.34):   Slowly lower your body as far as possible and then return to the starting position.

Precaution: This exercise should not be attempted if you have poor upper-body strength, as injury may occur in attempting to support your weight when returning to the starting position.

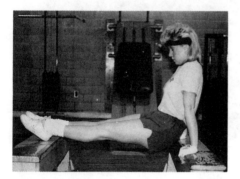

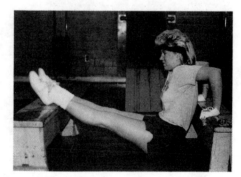

Figure 5.33

Figure 5.34

Curl-Ups

Major muscle groups: Abdominals (stomach).

Starting position: Lie in a supine position on the floor, with your upper legs held perpendicular to the floor. Bend your knees comfortably, cross your ankles, and cross your hands across your chest or place your hands along side of your head for resistance. *Do not pull your hands against your head or neck.*

Movement (Figure 5.35):   Keeping the legs stationary, raise your trunk no more than 30 to 45 degrees from the floor to prevent possible lower-back injury. Then return to the starting position.

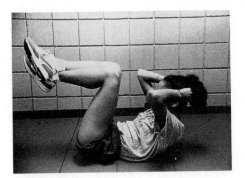

Figure 5.35

CIRCUIT TRAINING

Due to the nature of resistance training—that is, short periods of exercise of moderate-to-intense exertion followed by rest periods—essentially no cardiorespiratory conditioning occurs. Circuit training is a method of exercise that conditions both the muscular and cardiorespiratory systems of the body. The term **circuit** refers to a number of carefully selected exercises, called **stations,** arranged in a "circuit" and performed in a prescribed sequence. This sequence permits the exerciser to engage in continuous activity by moving from one station to the next without pausing to rest. Progression on a circuit occurs by decreasing the time required to traverse the entire circuit, increasing the amount of exercise performed at the various stations, or a combination of both.

A distinctive feature of circuit training is its adaptability to a number of situations. For example, a program developed for college-age men can easily be modified for other age groups or women. Circuits can be established both indoors and outdoors and can be shortened or lengthened to fit almost any time requirement. If the physical demands of a sport are known, a circuit can be developed that includes skill stations as well as weight training and calisthenic stations that will develop the muscles used in that particular sport. A circuit training program should be intense enough to maintain your heart rate in the target heart rate zone.

An innovation in circuit training is a cross-country circuit training course called a **parcourse.** A parcourse consists of several exercise stations located along a jogging trail. As you jog along the trail and arrive at an exercise station, a sign indicates the type of exercise and the **par**, or number of repetitions, to be performed before jogging to the next exercise station. Typical exercises performed along a parcourse include push-ups, pull-ups, sit-ups, and a variety of calisthenic-type stretching exercises.

Circuit Training Considerations.

In most cases exercisers perform a complete circuit three times. The number of repetitions, amount of resistance used, and speed of performance over the entire circuit determines the workload. Workload, also known as **exercise dosage**, should not be so intense that you are completely exhausted after completing the first lap of the circuit. On the other hand, it must be sufficiently challenging to require performance near maximal capacity during the final lap.

Before you engage in high-intensity circuit training, determine the proper exercise dosage for each station in the circuit. The recommended method is to spend the first day on the circuit evaluating yourself on each exercise in the circuit. Do this by performing the *maximum* number of repetitions for each exercise in the same order that they appear in the circuit, with a one- or two-minute rest between exercises. Starting exercise dosage is usually set at *half* the maximum number of repetitions performed. For example, if pull-ups are an exercise in the circuit and you can perform ten, the exercise dosage should be set at five.

In setting exercise dosages for muscular-endurance exercises such as bent-knee sit-ups where 50 or more repetitions are possible, it is best to evaluate maximum performance within a specified time period, usually 30 to 60 seconds. Again, starting exercise dosage should be *half* the repetitions performed within the time limit. For example, if you can perform 25 situps in 30, set the exercise dosage at 12 or 13.

When running is included in a circuit, the minimum time required to traverse a specified distance is *doubled* to set a reasonable exercise dosage. For example, if you can run a quarter-mile in one minute, set the exercise dosage at two minutes.

Once you establish exercise dosages and total time for completing the circuit, you can set new goals as you gain strength and endurance. Generally, it is more convenient to keep the completion time constant and to progress by increasing the exercise dosage at the various stations. If barbells are available, you can substitute or add weight training exercises to the circuit. In setting exercise dosages for weight training exercises, the recommended resistance should be approximately *three-quarters* of your ten-repetition maximal load. Thus, if you can upright-curl eighty pounds, ten times, you would set the exercise dosage to be ten repetitions at sixty pounds.

Following are examples of typical circuit training programs. Program #1 is less intensive and is basically a calisthenic-type exercise circuit. The second program is considerably more intensive and includes calisthenics, running, and weight training.

Circuit Training Program #1

STATION	EXERCISE	EVALUATION	MAXIMUM PERFORMANCE	EXERCISE DOSAGE
1	Side-straddle hops	Maximum in 30 seconds		
2	Push-ups	Maximum		
3	Cross-over curl-ups	Maximum in 30 seconds		
4	Running in place	Maximum in 30 seconds		
5	Pull-ups	Maximum		
6	Alternate toe-touches curl-ups	Maximum in 30 seconds		

Circuit Training Program #2

STATION	EXERCISE	EVALUATION	MAXIMUM PERFORMANCE	EXERCISE DOSAGE
1	Run/jog 440 yards	Minimum time		
2	Bent-knee sit-ups	Maximum in 30 secs		
3	Upright curls	Maximum wt., 10 reps.		
4	Run/jog 440 yards	Minimum time		
5	Prone back-lift	Maximum in 30 secs.		
6	Upright press	Maximum wt., 10 reps.		
7	Run/jog 440 yards	Minimum time		
8	Upright row	Maximum wt., 10 reps.		
9	Half-squat, heel raised	Maximum wt., 15 reps.		
10	Run/jog 440 yards	Minimum time		
11	Hanging leg-raise	Maximum wt., 30 secs.		
12	Supine press	Maximum wt., 10 reps.		

SUPPLEMENTARY READINGS

Allen, E., R. Byrd, and D. Smith. "Hemodynamic Consequences of Circuit Weight Training." *Research Quarterly,* Vol. 47, No. 3, pp. 299–305, 1973.

Allsen, P. E., J. M. Harrison, and B. Vance. *Fitness for Life: An Individualized Approach.* 5th ed. Madison, WI: Brown & Benchmark, 1993.

Corbin, C. B., and R. Lindsey. *Concepts of Physical Fitness with Laboratories.* 8th ed. Madison, WI: Brown & Benchmark, 1994.

Darden, E. *The Nautilus Book.* Chicago: Contemporary Books, 1990.

Dobbins, B. *High Tech Training.* New York: Simon and Schuster, 1982.

Getchell, B. *Physical Fitness: A Way of Life.* 4th ed. New York: Macmillan, 1992.

Gettman, L., L. Calter, and T. Strathman. "Physiologic Changes After 20 Weeks of Isotonic vs. Isokinetic Circuit Training." *Journal of Sports Medicine and Physical Fitness,* Vol. 20, No. 3, 1980.

Hesson, J. L. *Weight Training.* 3d ed. Englewood, CO: Morton Publishing, 1995.

Knuttgen, H. G. "Force, Work, Power and Exercise." *Medicine and Science in Sports,* Vol. 10, No. 3, pp. 227–228, 1978.

Rasch, P. J. *Weight Training.* 5th ed. Madison, WI: Brown & Benchmark, 1990.

Roskamm, H. "Optimum Patterns of Exercise for Healthy Men." *Canadian Medical Association Journal,* Vol. 67, pp. 895–899, 1967.

Westcott, W. L. *Strength Fitness: Physiological Principles and Training Techniques.* 4th ed. Madison, WI: Brown & Benchmark, 1994.

CHAPTER 5 REVIEW QUESTIONS

1. List five benefits of a muscular-strength-and-endurance training program.

    a.

    b.

    c.

    d.

    e.

2. List three types of muscular contraction.

    a.

    b.

    c.

3. List three genetic factors that affect physical performance.

    a.

    b.

    c.

4. What accounts for the muscular hypertrophy and strength differences between men and women?

5. Women and older men apparently gain strength by:

6. What is progressive-resistance exercise?

7. What is isotonic training?

8. What is isometric training?

9. What is isokinetic training?

10. Define the following:
    a. repetition:

    b. set:

    c. sticking point:

11. What is the "Valsalva phenomenon" and how can you prevent it?

12. What precautions should you take when lifting a barbell from the floor?

13. Why should you use good form when lifting weights?

14. List three things that help avoid muscle-boundness.

    a.

    b.

    c.

15. Total-body development is necessary to:

    a.

    b.

16. How does periodically varying some of the exercises in your workout program increase the overall strength of a muscle group?

17. The sequence for exercising should progress from _____ to _____ muscle groups.

18. If your time is limited, your workout should comprise exercises that develop which muscles?

19. What are some general guidelines regarding training frequency, intensity, and time?

    a. frequency:

    b. intensity:

    c. time:

20. List six training systems used in weight training.

 a.

 b.

 c.

 d.

 e.

 f.

21. When should you use spotters in weight training?

22. What is circuit training?

23. How should you determine your exercise dosage?

CHAPTER

6

Nutrition and Health

The complex biological makeup of the human body requires consuming a proper diet in order to have energy, regenerate cells, and maintain physiological homeostasis. "You are what you eat" is taking on new meaning as fast-food outlets take in more and more of our food dollars. Some experts believe that the eating habits of the American people have never been worse.

Nutrition has a significant effect on health. It contributes to virtually every function of your body. Nutrients from food are necessary for every heartbeat, nerve sensation, and muscle contraction. Good nutrition not only prevents deficiency diseases such as scurvy and anemia, but also improves resistance to infectious diseases and plays a role in the prevention of chronic diseases. Good nutrition is preventive medicine.

THE NUTRIENTS

Nutrition is easy to understand if we keep the volume of information in a simple and logical pattern. There are six basic classifications of nutrients. Each nutrient is vital to good health. A deficiency in any of these areas will alter your body's dietary balance. The classifications are

1. carbohydrates
2. proteins
3. fats
4. vitamins
5. minerals
6. water

Carbohydrates, proteins, and fats provide energy by way of cellular metabolism. A measure of metabolic rate in units of heat is represented by a **calorie.** A calorie represents the heat required to raise 1 gram of water 1 degree Celsius. One Calorie (with a capital *C*), or kilocalorie, is equivalent to 1,000 calories. Approximately 3,500 kilocalories (Kcals) will equal one pound of body weight. The average adult male needs approximately 2,700 kcals per day while the average adult female requires about 2,100 kcals. These values may increase or decrease depending upon the activity level of the individual. Vitamins, minerals, and water are important in the metabolic process but do not provide calories.

NUTRIENT	GRAMS	CALORIES
carbohydrate	1	4
protein	1	4
fat	1	9

Carbohydrates. Carbohydrates (CHO) are our body's primary source of energy. They will comprise between 45 to 70 percent of your daily caloric intake. The word *carbohydrate* is derived from its organic structure—a pattern of carbon, hydrogen, and oxygen ($C_6 H_{12} O_6$). While the simple (**monosaccharide**) structure remains the same, carbohydrates can take different forms, such as double sugars (**disaccharides,** two simple sugars hooked together) and complex sugars (**polysaccharides,** more than two simple sugars). Examples of each type are

simple sugars:	glucose, fructose (fruit), galactose
double sugars:	sucrose (table sugar), maltose
complex sugars:	starch (grains), cellulose (fiber)

Digestion of disaccharides and polysaccharides will produce glucose, a major source of energy for the working muscles. When glucose enters the bloodstream, your body will use it in one of three ways:

1. *Energy production,* if your body needs the fuel; if one gram of carbohydrate is synthesized, four Calories (kilocalories) will be produced
2. *Storage as glycogen (glycogenesis),* if your liver and muscles are not already saturated with glycogen
3. *Conversion to fat,* if cells can store no more glycogen

Carbohydrates supply about 50 percent of your body's energy at rest and, during high-intensity exercise, this percentage increases in order to sustain the activity. Energy from carbohydrates can be produced **anaerobically** (without oxygen) or **aerobically** (with oxygen). Thus, carbohydrates release energy faster than fats but for a shorter period of time.

Complex carbohydrates are more nutritious and are digested more efficiently than refined sugars; they should therefore comprise the majority of your CHO intake. A diet high in complex carbohydrates tends to lessen the insulin response that occurs after eating, as compared to a diet high in refined sugars. You can improve your diet by determining which foods contain refined sugars and replacing them with simple sugars (fruits) and complex sugars (grain products). You may ask "What is the benefit of substituting an apple for a candy bar? Aren't they both sugars?" It is not that the apple is a "perfect" food, but it does not contain the fat, refined sugar, and calories of the candy bar. Therefore, the benefit is in what you avoid in the candy bar (fat, refined sugar, and calories) and what you gain from the fruit (nutrients, fiber, and fewer calories).

Fats. Fats function as a carrier for fat-soluble vitamins, serve as an insulator and body-temperature regulator, and can also provide a large amount of energy. A molecule of fat has the identical structural components of a carbohydrate. However, the arrangement of these atoms differs in that the hydrogen count exceeds the oxygen count in a fat molecule. Of the two types of dietary fats, one fatty acid, *saturated*, has a single bond between the carbon atoms. The other, *unsaturated,* has a double bond between the carbon atoms. This difference reduces the potential for unsaturated fatty acids to bind with hydrogen. Unsaturated fats are easier to convert into short carbon chains than saturated fats are. Therefore, nutritionists recommend that unsaturated fats be consumed in a 2:1 ratio to saturated fats. Diets high in saturated fat contribute to atherosclerosis (plaque in arteries).

Fats are initially broken down in the small intestine. Once fat enters the bloodstream, the enzyme lipoprotein lipase converts the fat into fatty acids that are used for energy synthesis or stored as triglycerides in adipose tissue. If needed, the stored fat can be removed from the adipose cells and used as energy. One gram of fat will yield nine calories of energy.

The typical American diet consists of an unacceptable amount of fat, particularly saturated fat. Many people consume 35 to 40 percent of their daily calorie total in the form of fat. This is too high. Your body will adapt quite nicely if these percentages are reduced to 15 to 20 percent with the majority being unsaturated. However, the average American may have a difficult time reaching this level simply because of a traditional preference for foods high in fat. A positive step in lowering the saturated-fat content of your diet is to identify the high-risk foods and attempt to substitute foods lower in fat.

A critical factor in the fat content of many foods involves the preparation. A classic example is fried foods—many nutritious foods are altered by the tendency to fry with animal and vegetable oils that are usually 100 percent fat.

Some primary sources of fats are red meats, butter, cheese, cream, and peanuts. Table 6.1 lists various sources of saturated and unsaturated fats. Table 6.2 classifies some of the common dietary oils.

As mentioned in Chapter 4, undesirable cholesterol levels can have an adverse effect on your cardiorespiratory health. Your diet can influence these levels. You should know the factors that have the greatest impact upon your cholesterol level. They are

1. dietary fat
2. dietary cholesterol
3. dietary fiber

Dietary fat has the largest single effect upon your cholesterol level. Doctors recommend keeping dietary fat below 30 percent of your daily caloric intake. You ingest dietary cholesterol when you consume foods of animal origin. Since white meat and fish generally contain less cholesterol than red meats, reduce your red meat intake by consuming more white meat and fish. Also, replace whole-milk dairy products that are high in fat with low-fat dairy products. Your dietary-fiber consumption should be 25 to 40 grams per day. If your fiber intake is currently low, slowly increase your daily consumption until you reach the desired level. A sudden change in daily fiber consumption will not allow your body to properly adjust to the increased "bulk" in your gastrointestinal tract.

Proteins.   Proteins are complex molecules containing amino acids. They serve the following functions:

1. cellular growth and repair
2. enzyme production
3. energy
4. blood sugar conversion
5. fat conversion

Table 6.1 Common sources of fat.

FOOD	PERCENT FAT	PERCENT SATURATED	PERCENT UNSATURATED
Animal Sources			
Beef	16–42	52	48
Chicken	10–17	30	70
Beef heart	6	50	50
Lamb	19–29	60	40
Ham, sliced	23	45	55
Pork	32	45	55
Veal cutlet	10	50	50
Butter	81	55	36
Plant Sources			
Cashew nuts	48	18	82
Peanut butter	50	25	75
Carrots	0	0	0
Potato chips	35	25	75
Margarine	81	26	66
Corn oil	100	7	78
Cottonseed oil	100	21.5	71.5
Olive oil	100	14	86
Soybean oil	100	14	71.5

Reprinted by permission from McArdle, W.D., Katch, F.I., and Katch, V.L. *Exercise Physiology: Nutrition and Human Performance*. Philadelphia: Lea & Febiger, 1986.

Table 6.2 Classification of common dietary oils.

Saturated	red meats, palm, coconut, palm kernel
Unsaturated	
(Mono)	avocado, canola, olive, peanut
(Poly)	corn, soybean, sunflower

Nine of the 20 amino acids needed by the body cannot be synthesized by your body and must be obtained through your diet; these nine are therefore termed the "essential" amino acids. Although all amino acids are used primarily for cellular growth and repair, they can be converted to blood sugar for energy, or they can be converted to and stored as fat if the carbohydrate stores are saturated. If used for energy, one gram of protein yields four calories of energy.

The recommended daily allowance (RDA) of protein for adults is a minimum of .4 gram per kilogram of body weight. The ideal intake is .9 gram per kilogram of body weight. For infants and growing children, the RDA is 2.0 and 4.0 grams per kilogram of body weight, respectively. Protein should constitute 15 to 20 percent of your daily caloric total.

Proteins that contain the essential amino acids can be consumed from plant and animal cells. *Complete proteins* contain all the essential amino acids in quality and quantity for nitrogen balance, tissue growth, and tissue repair. *Incomplete proteins* lack one or more of the essential amino acids. Quality protein foods (complete proteins) are usually of animal origin, such as eggs, meat, fish, poultry, and milk. However, most complete proteins are high in cholesterol, which increases the risk for coronary heart disease. Lower-quality (incomplete) protein sources are mostly of vegetable origin, such as beans, peas, nuts, and breads. Through careful planning you can combine a variety of the incomplete protein foods to meet the RDA for all essential amino acids without having to consume foods high in cholesterol.

Vitamins.   Vitamins are essential for controlling bodily functions such as regulating metabolic reactions for energy synthesis. Some vitamins (A, D, E, and K) are fat-soluble and can be stored in the body. Vitamins B and C are water-soluble and must be ingested on a daily basis. See Table 6.3 for the functions and sources of each vitamin.

Minerals.   The most valuable function of minerals is regulation of cellular metabolism. Minerals are classified as major and trace minerals. Table 6.4 lists the sources and functions of essential minerals.

Water.   The body contains water in extracellular (outside the cell) and intracellular (inside the cell) areas. Blood, saliva, fluids from glands and the intestines, and fluids excreted from the skin are extracellular areas high in water content. Water is a vital element in bodily functions even though it does not actually contribute to the nutritional value of food. Water comprises approximately 60 percent of your body weight and acts as a transfer medium for vital bodily processes. It also aids in body-temperature regulation.

The typical adult requires approximately 2.5 liters of water every day. Large quantities of water are excreted as urine and bodily waste, while smaller amounts are lost in respiration and cellular metabolism. Water loss from exercise varies from individual to individual. In general, the warmer the environment is, the more an individual will need to perspire in order to aid the body in temperature regulation. Consequently, this elevates the body's need to replenish its water stores. You usually satisfy your thirst for water before properly replenishing the body's stores. Therefore, you should "force" yourself to drink extra liquids, especially after exercising in the heat. As a general rule, you should replenish *each pound* of body weight lost through sweat with *one pint* of fluid. Don't attempt to rehydrate with one giant gulp, but do drink often enough to balance your water loss within 30 to 45 minutes after exercising. Water is usually sufficient to rehydrate your body. If your activity lasted more than 45 to 60 minutes, it may also be beneficial to include a replacement drink that contains sodium—the electrolyte most depleted in sweat loss—and some form of carbohydrate (glucose, fructose) to provide energy for the working muscles and to stimulate fluid absorption in the gastrointestinal tract. Commercial fluid replacement beverages that taste good usually encourage more intake by a dehydrated exerciser.

NUTRITION GUIDELINES

Since the typical American diet is inadequate to maintain optimal health and freedom from disease, the U.S. Senate Committee on Nutrition and Human Needs has endorsed the *Prudent Diet* to assist you in your daily eating habits. This committee, with recommendations from nutrition and food experts, established the seven dietary goals listed on page 88–89.

Table 6.3   Major sources and functions of vitamins.

NUTRIENT	GOOD SOURCES	MAJOR FUNCTIONS	DEFICIENCY SYMPTOMS
Vitamin A	Milk, cheese, butter, fortified margarine, eggs, liver, and orange/yellow/dark green fruits and vegetables.	Required for healthy bones, teeth, skin, gums, and hair. Maintenance of inner mucous membranes, thus increasing resistance to infection. Adequate vision in dim light.	Night blindness, decreased growth, decreased resistance to infection, rough or dry skin.
Vitamin D	Fortified milk, cod liver oil, salmon, tuna, and egg yolks.	Necessary for bones and teeth. Needed for calcium and phosphorous absorption.	Rickets (bone softening), fractures, and muscle spasms.
Vitamin E	Vegetable oils, yellow and green leafy vegetables, margarine, wheat germ, and whole grain breads and cereals.	Related to oxidation and normal muscle and red blood cell chemistry.	Leg cramps, red blood cell breakdown.
Vitamin K	Green leafy vegetables, cauliflower, cabbage, eggs, peas, and potatoes.	Essential for normal blood clotting.	Hemorrhaging.
Vitamin B1 (Thiamine)	Enriched bread, lean meat, fish, liver, pork, poultry, organ meats, legumes, nuts, dried yeast, and milk.	Assists in proper use of carbohydrates, normal functioning of nervous system, and maintenance of good appetite.	Loss of appetite, nausea, confusion, cardiac abnormalities, muscle spasms.
Vitamin B2 (Riboflavin)	Eggs, milk, leafy green vegetables,whole grains, lean meats, and dried beans and peas.	Contributes to energy release from carbohydrates, fats, and proteins. Needed for normal growth and development, good vision, and healthy skin.	Cracking of the corners of the mouth, inflammation of the skin, impaired vision.
Vitamin B6 (Pyridoxine)	Vegetables, meats, whole-grain cereals, soybeans, peanuts, and potatoes.	Necessary for protein and fatty acid metabolism, and normal red blood cell formation.	Depression, irritability, muscle spasms, nausea.

(continued)

Table 6.3 Continued.

NUTRIENT	GOOD SOURCES	MAJOR FUNCTIONS	DEFICIENCY SYMPTOMS
Vitamin B12	Meat, poultry, fish, liver, organ meats, eggs, shellfish, milk, and cheese.	Required for normal growth, red blood cell formation, nervous system and digestive tract functioning.	Impaired balance, weakness, drop in red blood cell count.
Niacin	Liver and organ meats, meat, fish, poultry, whole grains, enriched breads, nuts, green leafy vegetables, and dried beans and peas.	Contributes to energy release from carbohydrates, fats, and proteins. Normal growth and development and formation of hormones and nerve-regulating substances.	Confusion, depression, weakness, weight loss.
Biotin	Liver, kidney, eggs, yeast, legumes, milk, nuts, and dark green vegetables.	Essential for carbohydrate metabolism and fatty acid synthesis.	Inflamed skin, muscle pain, depression, weight loss.
Folic Acid	Leafy green vegetables, organ meats, whole grains and cereals, and dried beans.	Needed for cell growth and reproduction and red blood cell formation.	Decreased resistance to infection.
Pantothenic Acid	All natural foods, especially liver, kidney, eggs, nuts, yeast, milk, dried peas and beans, and green leafy vegetables.	Related to carbohydrate and fat metabolism.	Depression, low blood sugar, leg cramps, nausea, headaches.
Vitamin C (Ascorbic Acid)	Fruits and vegetables.	Helps protect against infection. Aids formation of collagenous tissue, normal blood vessels, teeth, and bones.	Slow-healing wounds, loose teeth, hemorrhaging, rough or scaly skin, irritability.

From *Lifetime Physical Fitness and Wellness: A Personalized Program* by Werner W. K. Hoeger. Copyright © 1988 by Morton Publishing, Englewood, CO. Used with permission.

Table 6.4   Major sources and functions of minerals.

NUTRIENT	GOOD SOURCES	MAJOR FUNCTIONS	DEFICIENCY SYMPTOMS
Calcium	Milk, cheese, green leafy vegetables, dried beans, sardines, salmon, and citrus fruits.	Required for strong teeth and bone formation. Maintenance of good muscle tone, heartbeat, and nerve function.	Bone pain and fractures, periodontal disease, muscle cramps.
Iron	Organ meats, lean meats, seafoods, eggs, dried peas and beans, nuts, whole and enriched grains, and green leafy vegetables.	Major component of hemoglobin. Aids in energy utilization.	Nutritional anemia and overall weakness.
Phosphorus	Meats, fish, milk, eggs, dried beans and peas, whole grains, and processed foods.	Required for bone and teeth formation. Energy-release regulation.	Bone pain and fractures, weight loss, and weakness.
Zinc	Milk, meat, seafood, whole grains, nuts, eggs, and dried beans.	Essential component of hormones, insulin, and enzymes. Used in normal growth and development.	Loss of appetite, slow-healing wounds, and skin problems.
Magnesium	Green leafy vegetables, whole grains, nuts, soybeans, seafood, and legumes.	Needed for bone growth and maintenance, carbohydrate and protein utilization, nerve function, and temperature regulation.	Irregular heartbeat, weakness, muscle spasms, and sleeplessness.
Sodium	Table salt, processed foods, and meat.	Body-fluid regulation. Transmission of nerve impulses. Heart action.	Rarely seen.
Potassium	Legumes, whole grains, bananas, orange juice, dried fruits, and potatoes.	Heart action. Bone formation and maintenance. Regulation of energy release. Acid–base regulation.	Irregular heartbeat, nausea, and weakness.

From *Lifetime Physical Fitness and Wellness: A Personalized Program* by Werner W. K. Hoeger. Copyright © 1988 by Morton Publishing, Englewood, CO. Used with permission.,

1. To avoid overweightness, balance the caloric intake with the caloric expenditure; if overweight, decrease the caloric intake and increase the caloric expenditure.

2. Increase the consumption of complex carbohydrates and *naturally occurring* sugars.

3. Reduce the consumption of refined and processed sugars.
4. Reduce the total consumption of fats.
5. Reduce saturated fat consumption and balance that with polyunsaturated and monoun-saturated fats.
6. Reduce cholesterol consumption to about 300 milligrams per day.
7. Limit the intake of sodium by reducing the intake of salt to about five grams per day (the equivalent of one teaspoon).

Nutritionists view these changes in your diet as beneficial in reducing the risk of chronic diseases (such as heart disease and diabetes) that plague modern society. You can effect these changes by

1. increasing your consumption of fruits, vegetables, and whole grains
2. decreasing your consumption of red meat and increasing your consumption of poultry and fish
3. decreasing your consumption of foods high in fat and partially substituting polyunsaturated for saturated fat
4. substituting nonfat milk for whole milk
5. decreasing your consumption of butterfat, eggs, and other high-cholesterol sources
6. decreasing your consumption of sugar and foods with high sugar content
7. decreasing your consumption of salt and foods with high salt content

The *Food Pyramid* (see Figure 6.1), released by the U. S. Department of Agriculture in 1992, will help you reach the goals of the Prudent Diet. The Food Pyramid divides food into six groups and recommends the number of daily servings from each group. The shape of the pyramid indicates how much of the food group you should eat: foods at the wide base of the pyramid should make up the largest portion of your diet while the foods at the tip should be eaten infrequently.

If you are interested in determining the percentage of fats, carbohydrates, and other nutrients in your diet, begin by reading the food labels now required on nearly all packaged foods. See Figure 6.2 for a brief explanation of the new food label.

Figure 6.1   The Food Pyramid.

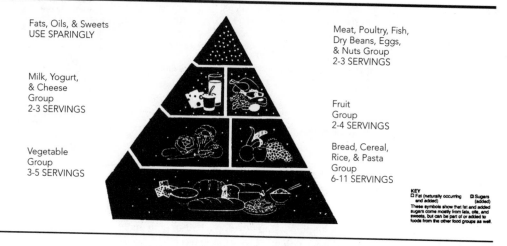

Figure 6.2   Using the new food label.

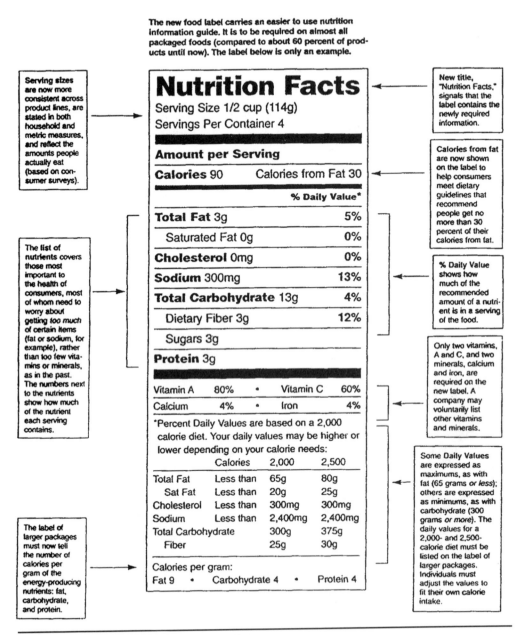

The new food label carries an easier to use nutrition information guide. It is to be required on almost all packaged foods (compared to about 60 percent of products until now). The label below is only an example.

Serving sizes are now more consistent across product lines, are stated in both household and metric measures, and reflect the amounts people actually eat (based on consumer surveys).

New title, "Nutrition Facts," signals that the label contains the newly required information.

Nutrition Facts

Serving Size 1/2 cup (114g)
Servings Per Container 4

Amount per Serving

| **Calories** 90 | Calories from Fat 30 |

Calories from fat are now shown on the label to help consumers meet dietary guidelines that recommend people get no more than 30 percent of their calories from fat.

% **Daily Value***

Total Fat 3g	5%
Saturated Fat 0g	0%
Cholesterol 0mg	0%
Sodium 300mg	13%
Total Carbohydrate 13g	4%
Dietary Fiber 3g	12%
Sugars 3g	
Protein 3g	

The list of nutrients covers those most important to the health of consumers, most of whom need to worry about getting *too much* of certain items (fat or sodium, for example), rather than too few vitamins or minerals, as in the past. The numbers next to the nutrients show how much of the nutrient each serving contains.

% Daily Value shows how much of the recommended amount of a nutrient is in a serving of the food.

Vitamin A	80%	•	Vitamin C	60%
Calcium	4%	•	Iron	4%

*Percent Daily Values are based on a 2,000 calorie diet. Your daily values may be higher or lower depending on your calorie needs:

Only two vitamins, A and C, and two minerals, calcium and iron, are required on the new label. A company may voluntarily list other vitamins and minerals.

	Calories	2,000	2,500
Total Fat	Less than	65g	80g
Sat Fat	Less than	20g	25g
Cholesterol	Less than	300mg	300mg
Sodium	Less than	2,400mg	2,400mg
Total Carbohydrate		300g	375g
Fiber		25g	30g

Calories per gram:
Fat 9   •   Carbohydrate 4   •   Protein 4

The label of larger packages must now tell the number of calories per gram of the energy-producing nutrients: fat, carbohydrate, and protein.

Some Daily Values are expressed as maximums, as with fat (65 grams *or less*); others are expressed as minimums, as with carbohydrate (300 grams *or more*). The daily values for a 2,000- and 2,500-calorie diet must be listed on the label of larger packages. Individuals must adjust the values to fit their own calorie intake.

Source: U. S. Food and Drug Administration, 1993.

ALCOHOL

Abstention from or prudent use of alcoholic beverages is an individual responsibility. If you decide to drink alcohol, it is important that you develop a responsible pattern of behavior that you can follow for a lifetime; in addition, you need to understand some basic facts regarding its use.

Alcohol is a depressant and therefore slows the mental and physical functions of the body. These functions include memory recall, cognitive thinking, reaction time, strength, and skills involving fine motor movement patterns. It has been estimated that over 50 percent of all fatal traffic accidents involve a drinking driver. In addition, alcoholic beverages are high in calories but low in nutrients; this means heavy drinkers often have problems with overfatness and nutrition, since they tend to allow alcohol to displace more nutritious foods in their diets. It is common knowledge that heavy alcohol use causes cirrhosis of the liver. Also, evidence now supports the concept that drinking alcohol during a pregnancy may cause permanent damage to the baby.

Not drinking alcohol will not detract from the happiness in your life, but irresponsible drinking will lead to a drinking problem. When a drinking problem exists, its negative effects rarely harm only the drinker. It also affects friends, family members, and others who come into contact with the drinker.

Your tolerance or lack of tolerance for alcohol depends upon many things, including an empty stomach, mood and attitude, food consumption, illness, physical problems such as diabetes, heredity, and the amount and type of beverage consumed. In addition, the faster you drink, the faster the alcohol reaches the bloodstream. Therefore, if you do drink, the beverage should be sipped, not gulped. Finally, the lower your body weight, the higher the blood alcohol level for a given amount of alcohol consumed.

Information concerning drinking and its related problems is available at most student health and counseling services. Be smart! Don't let alcohol mess up an enjoyable life.

COMMONLY ASKED QUESTIONS ABOUT NUTRITION

Following are common questions concerning diet and fitness:

1. *Why are whole grains better than refined grains?*

   Trace amounts of minerals, vitamin B, and other nutrients are removed during the refining process. The enrichment process adds back some of these nutrients, but whole grains contain more fiber and nutrients than refined grains do.

2. *When training intensively, should individuals increase their intake of protein?*

   Yes, but only for the first week. Apparently, the initiation of an intensive training program causes individuals on a diet containing "normal" amounts of protein (.9 grams per kilogram of body weight) to go into negative nitrogen balance (net loss of protein). During the first week of training, the protein intake should be increased to 1.5 grams per kilogram of body weight. After the first week, the normal recommended amount of .9 grams per kilogram of body weight appears to be sufficient.

3. *Does sugar consumption in the form of candy or soda before an exercise event provide quick energy?*

   Sugar consumption before an exercise event results in an insulin reaction; blood sugar (glucose) is removed from the blood, leaving you with less energy than you would have had without the sugar.

4. *Are vitamin and mineral supplements necessary?*

   The body generally cannot utilize additional quantities of any vitamin other than the amount required for normal function. As long as the diet provides adequate nutrients, supplementation does not help.

5. *What are the recommended daily allowances (RDA) of iron?*

   College-aged males should receive 10 milligrams per deciliter of blood (mg/d), while college-aged females should receive 15 mg/d.

6. *How many calories (Kcals) do I burn while doing some type of aerobic exercise?*

   A simple equation to remember is that you will burn a quantity of calories equal to your body weight for every 10 minutes of continuous aerobic exercise at a moderate intensity. If you weigh 150 pounds and jog for 30 minutes, you would burn approximately 450 Kcals (150 lbs. × 10 minutes × 3 = 450).

7. *How much time should I allow between eating and exercising?*

   Your working muscles perform best when the gastrointestinal (GI) tract is not attempting to digest a meal. During exercise, blood flow is diverted to the working muscles. If you are simultaneously trying to digest food, your GI tract will keep some of the blood for that process. Thus there is less energy available for the exercising muscles. Allow yourself at least two hours between eating and exercising. If you do eat just prior to exercise, the food should be easily digestible (fluids and/or light snack).

8. *What mineral plays an important part in bone development?*

   Calcium is the most critical mineral for bone development. The recommended daily calcium intake ranges from 400 mg (infants) to 1,200 mg (adults). Including a load-bearing activity on a regular basis (45 minutes three times per week) is also suggested to help promote bone growth and maintenance.

9. *What effect does caffeine have on endurance performance?*

   There have been few conclusive studies of the effects of caffeine on endurance performance. Caffeine has not been proven to enhance or hinder endurance performance.

SUPPLEMENTARY READINGS

Allsen, P. E., J. M. Harrison, and B. Vance. *Fitness for Life: An Individual Approach.* 5th ed. Madison, WI: Brown & Benchmark, 1993.

Dintiman, G. B., R. G. Davis, S. E. Stone, and J. C. Pennington. Ed. by Marshall. *Discovering Lifetime Fitness: Concepts of Exercise and Weight Control.* 2d ed. St. Paul, MN: West Publishing, 1989.

Ettinger, B., H. K. Genaut, and C. E. Cann. "Postmenopausal Bone Loss is Prevented by Treatment with Low-Dosage Estrogen with Calcium." *Annals of Internal Medicine.* Vol. 106, pp. 40–45, 1987.

Fox, E. L. *Lifetime Fitness.* Dubuque, IA: Wm. C. Brown, 1988.

McArdle, W. D., F. I. Katch, and V. L. Katch. *Exercise Physiology: Energy, Nutrition, and Human Performance.* 3d ed. Baltimore, MD: Williams & Wilkins, 1991.

McNaughton, L. "Two Levels of Caffeine Ingestion on Blood Lactate and Free Fatty Acid Responses During Incremental Exercise." *Research Quarterly for Exercise and Sport.* Vol. 58, pp. 255–259, 1987.

Prentice, W. E., et al. *Fitness for College and Life.* 4th ed. St. Louis, MO: Mosby–Year Book, 1993.

U.S. Senate Select Committee on Nutrition and Human Needs. *Dietary Goals for the United States.* Washington, DC: Government Printing Office, 1977.

CHAPTER 6 REVIEW QUESTIONS

1. What are the three categories of "energy" foods?

   a.

   b.

   c.

2. How do vitamins, minerals, and water function in the body?

3. Proteins are used for

   a.

   b.

   c.

   d.

   e.

4. What is meant by the term "essential amino acid"?

5. The recommended daily allowance of protein for adults is ideally _____ grams per kilogram of body weight.

6. What is a "complete" protein?

7. Protein should constitute _____ to _____ percent of your daily caloric total.

8. Three examples of simple carbohydrates include
   a.

   b.

   c.

9. Three examples of disaccharides include
   a.

   b.

   c.

10. Two forms of complex carbohydrates include
    a.

    b.

11. What are the three ways your body uses glucose?
    a.

    b.

    c.

12. Although carbohydrates comprise approximately _____ to _____ percent of the total calories in the typical American's diet, they really should comprise _____ to _____ percent of the total caloric intake.

13. Why is it better to eat an apple than a candy bar?

14. What is the difference between saturated and unsaturated fats?

15. Diets that are high in saturated fats contribute to:

16. Which dietary component has the largest single effect upon your cholesterol level?

17. It is recommended that which dietary component be kept below 30 percent of your daily caloric intake?

18. Dietary cholesterol is ingested by consuming foods of:

19. Dietary fiber consumption should be between _____ to _____ grams per day.

20. The typical adult requires approximately _____ liters of water every day.

21. What does it mean to "force" liquids?

22. What are the seven dietary goals of the Senate Committee on Nutrition and Human Needs?

    a.

    b.

    c.

    d.

    e.

    f.

    g.

23. List seven things you can do to reach the goals listed above.

    a.

    b.

    c.

    d.

    e.

    f.

    g.

24. What are some of the problems with alcohol consumption?

CHAPTER

7

Body Composition and Weight Control

Thirty to sixty percent of the American public are obese. However, obesity should be distinguished from being overweight as indicated by height-and-weight charts used by insurance companies. Excessive body weight may be due to an accumulation of body fat or muscle mass. For example, muscular men often have body weights that far exceed the norms for their height and weight and yet have a low percentage of body fat. Obesity is being *overfat,* not *overweight.*

The amount of fat accumulation on your body is commonly expressed as a percentage of your total body weight and is referred to as percent body fat. Table 7.1 classifies body composition based on percent body fat.

ASSESSMENT OF BODY FAT

Many methods can be used to estimate your body fat. Less accurate methods include pinching an inch, circumference measurements, and looking in the mirror. Although each of these methods does help, more accurate methods exist. Physiology labs normally use hydrostatic weighing and measurement of body volume, which is considered by the majority of experts to be the most accurate. However, this method is complex, time-consuming, space requiring, and expensive. Another method that correlates very well with hydrostatic weight and measurement of body volume is the use of skinfold measures. Using a set of skinfold calipers, the thickness of the skin is measured at various sites by gently grasping the skin between the thumb and index finger and drawing the skin away from the body. Normally the skinfold is drawn away from the body in the vertical plane; however, if the natural flow of the skin is in a diagonal or horizontal plane, the skinfold is measured in the appropriate natural plane. Table 7.2 lists percent body fat calculations for men using the sum of skinfold measures taken at the chest, abdomen, and thigh. Table 7.3 lists the sum of the measures for women taken at the arm, hip, and thigh.

Table 7.1   Body composition based on percent body fat.

	PERCENT BODY FAT	
CLASSIFICATION	MEN	WOMEN
Very lean	≤10	≤12
Lean	11–14	15–19
Average	15–18	20–24
Fat	19–23	25–31
Overfat (obese)	≥ 24	≥ 32

HAZARDS OF OBESITY

Physical appearance and social acceptance tend to be the dominant reasons that people become concerned with maintaining a normal body weight. Severe emotional and physical problems can occur from being overfat.

Emotional Problems.   Older children and adolescents are especially concerned about appearance and can suffer severe psychological maladjustments as a result of disfigurement caused by obesity. Overfat boys and girls are often subjected to ridicule and social rejection by their unthinking peers. The inferiority complexes and social withdrawals that often result from such nonacceptance can leave emotional scars that may remain with the overfat child throughout life.

Physical Problems.   As serious as the adverse effects of obesity on social and psychological well-being are, the destructive effects of obesity on physical health are even more pronounced. Obesity places an additional burden upon circulation and respiration, making the individual more susceptible to heart, lung, and blood-vessel disorders. Overfat individuals have less exercise tolerance, greater difficulty in normal breathing, and a higher frequency of respiratory infections than people with normal body-fat levels. Also, overfat individuals have greater risk for diabetes mellitus, high blood pressure, high cholesterol, kidney and gall bladder disease, and atherosclerosis. In general, medical statistics indicate the incidence of most diseases is greater in people who are overfat.

CAUSES OF OBESITY

Obesity occurs when your average daily caloric intake contains more calories than are needed to maintain body functions and meet the caloric expenditures of daily activities. Excess calories are stored in your body's fat cells in the form of adipose (fat) tissue and gradually increase fat weight to an undesirable amount. If you balance caloric intake with caloric expenditure, your body weight stabilizes and further increases in fat storage do not occur. Creating a negative caloric imbalance results in a reduction in body weight as your body "borrows" calories from its fat cells to make up the caloric deficit.

Many factors influence the control of body weight. Some of these factors are listed on the following page.

Genetic Predisposition + Activity + Eating Habits = Weight

metabolic rate	work	types of food	maintain
number and type of	leisure	quantities	lose
fat cells	exercise	location	gain
gender		attitudes	
moods			

Genetic Predisposition.

The average American becomes more sedentary during the adult years. This leads to a decrease in lean muscle tissue and a decline in the metabolic rate. If your caloric intake is not reduced as the metabolic rate decreases, creeping obesity will occur. Creeping obesity, a form of obesity that occurs slowly over a period of several years, tends to be offset by an active lifestyle.

Experts believe that the metabolic rate can be controlled in an attempt to maintain an ideal biological weight (the setpoint) by a body-weight-and-fat-regulating mechanism located in the hypothalamus of the brain. This ideal biological weight is different for each individual. Apparently, the mechanism responds to both calories and nutrients. When you restrict your caloric intake, your body attempts to maintain the present weight and fat by lowering the metabolic rate. Also, when you have not consumed sufficient amounts of certain nutrients, your appetite increases. This setpoint is considered one of the primary reasons some people have such a hard time losing weight without gaining it back. According to the setpoint theory, the key to controlling weight is to control the setpoint. Lowering the setpoint can be accomplished through any of the following: (1) exercise, (2) a diet high in complex carbohydrates, (3) nicotine, and (4) amphetamines. Since nicotine and amphetamines have a destructive effect upon the body, the most effective way to lower the setpoint is through exercise combined with a diet high in complex carbohydrates.

There are two types of fat cells in the body—yellow and brown. The yellow fat cells are predominant, constituting approximately 99 percent of the total fat cells in the body. The number of yellow fat cells can be altered by diet and exercise during infancy and adolescence. Excessive caloric intake tends to promote yellow fat cell production in the formative years which, in turn, determines the ability of the body to store fat throughout life. To curb this potential for unnecessary yellow fat cell production, preventive steps need to be taken at an early age through proper nutritional and exercise habits. In light of what is now known about yellow fat cell production, the saying "A fat baby is a healthy baby" seems inappropriate.

Brown fat cells contain a high amount of the iron-containing hemoglobin pigment found in red blood cells. Instead of storing fat, it is thought that brown fat cells have the capacity to produce as much as 25 to 50 percent of the body's heat by burning fat. The number of brown fat cells appears to be genetically determined and not affected by exercise or diet. The number of brown fat cells varies from individual to individual. This helps explain why some individuals simply do not gain weight.

Gender affects the distribution of fat that individuals accumulate. Typically, females accumulate body fat on inner thighs and hips, while men accumulate fat in the waist area. These areas are usually the initial accumulation areas and the areas where fat remains the longest during a reduction program.

Activity Levels.

In today's society, machines perform many of the physically demanding jobs of the past. This automation has caused us to develop a much more sedentary lifestyle than at any previous time in history. Even sedentary leisure activities have

Table 7.2   Percent fat* estimates for men using the sum of the chest, abdominal, and thigh skinfold measures.

MALE SUM OF SKINFOLDS (mm)	<23	TO 27	23 TO 32	28 TO 37	33 TO 42	38 TO 47	43 TO 52	53 TO 57	58 AND OVER
8–10	1.3	1.8	2.3	2.9	3.4	3.9	4.5	5.0	5.5
11–13	2.2	2.8	3.3	3.9	4.4	4.9	5.5	6.0	6.5
14–16	3.2	3.8	4.3	4.8	5.4	5.9	6.4	7.0	7.5
17–19	4.2	4.7	5.3	5.8	6.3	6.9	7.4	8.0	8.5
20–22	5.1	5.7	6.2	6.8	7.3	7.9	8.4	8.9	9.5
23–25	6.1	6.6	7.2	7.7	8.3	8.8	9.4	9.9	10.5
26–28	7.0	7.6	8.1	8.7	9.2	9.8	10.3	10.9	11.4
29–31	8.0	8.5	9.1	9.6	10.2	10.7	11.3	11.8	12.4
32–34	8.9	9.4	10.0	10.5	11.1	11.6	12.2	12.8	13.3
35–37	9.8	10.4	10.9	11.5	12.0	12.6	13.1	13.7	14.3
38–40	10.7	11.3	11.8	12.4	12.9	13.5	14.1	14.6	15.2
41–43	11.6	12.2	12.7	13.3	13.8	14.4	15.0	15.5	16.1
44–46	12.5	13.1	13.6	14.2	14.7	15.3	15.9	16.4	17.0
47–49	13.4	13.9	14.5	15.1	15.6	16.2	16.8	17.3	17.9
50–52	14.3	14.8	15.4	15.9	16.5	17.1	17.6	18.2	18.8
53–55	15.1	15.7	16.2	16.8	17.4	17.9	18.5	19.1	19.7
56–58	16.0	16.5	17.1	17.7	18.2	18.8	19.4	20.0	20.5
59–61	16.9	17.4	17.9	18.5	19.1	19.7	20.2	20.8	21.4
62–64	17.6	18.2	18.8	19.4	19.9	20.5	21.1	21.7	22.2
65–67	18.5	19.0	19.6	20.2	20.8	21.3	21.9	22.5	23.1
68–70	19.3	19.9	20.4	21.0	21.6	22.2	22.7	23.3	23.9
71–73	20.1	20.7	21.2	21.8	22.4	23.0	23.6	24.1	24.7
74–76	20.9	21.5	22.0	22.6	23.2	23.8	24.4	25.0	25.5
77–79	21.7	22.2	22.8	23.4	24.0	24.6	25.2	25.8	26.3
80–82	22.4	23.0	23.6	24.2	24.8	25.4	25.9	26.5	27.1
83–85	23.4	23.8	24.4	25.0	25.5	26.1	26.7	27.3	27.9
86–88	24.0	24.5	25.1	25.7	26.3	26.9	27.5	28.1	28.7
89–91	24.7	25.3	26.9	25.5	27.1	27.6	28.2	28.8	29.4
92–94	25.4	26.0	26.6	27.2	27.8	28.4	29.0	29.6	30.2
95–97	26.1	26.7	27.3	27.9	28.5	29.1	29.7	30.3	30.9
98–100	26.9	27.4	28.0	28.6	29.2	29.8	30.4	31.0	31.6
101–103	27.5	28.1	28.7	29.3	29.9	30.5	31.1	31.7	32.3
104–106	28.2	28.8	29.4	30.0	30.6	31.2	31.8	32.4	33.0
107–109	28.9	29.5	30.1	30.7	31.3	31.9	32.5	33.1	33.7
110–112	29.6	30.2	30.8	31.4	32.0	32.6	33.2	33.8	34.4
113–115	30.2	30.8	31.4	32.0	32.6	33.2	33.8	34.5	35.1

*Percent fat calculated by the Siri Formula: (% fat = $[4.95 \div BD - 4.5] \times 100$), where BD = body density.

Taken from Pollock, M. L., Schmidt, D. H., and Jackson, A. S. "Measurement of Cardiorespiration Fitness and Body Composition in the Clinical Setting." *Comprehensive Therapy,* Vol. 6, September 1980.

Table 7.3 Percent fat* estimates for women using the sum of the triceps, iliac crest, and thigh skinfold measures.

FEMALE SUM OF SKINFOLDS (mm)	<23	TO 27	23 TO 32	28 TO 37	33 TO 42	38 TO 47	43 TO 52	53 TO 57	58 AND OVER
23–25	9.7	9.9	10.2	10.4	10.7	10.9	11.2	11.4	11.7
26–28	11.0	11.2	11.5	11.7	12.0	12.3	12.5	12.7	13.0
29–31	12.3	12.5	12.8	13.0	13.3	13.5	13.8	14.0	14.3
32–34	13.6	13.8	14.0	14.3	14.5	14.8	15.0	15.3	15.5
35–37	14.8	15.0	15.3	15.5	15.8	16.0	16.3	16.5	16.8
38–40	16.0	16.3	16.5	16.7	17.0	17.2	17.5	17.7	18.0
41–43	17.2	17.4	17.7	17.9	18.2	18.4	18.7	18.9	19.2
44–46	18.3	18.6	18.8	19.1	19.3	19.6	19.8	20.1	20.3
47–49	19.5	19.7	20.0	20.2	20.5	20.7	21.0	21.2	21.5
50–52	20.6	20.8	21.1	21.3	21.6	21.8	22.1	22.3	22.6
53–55	21.7	21.9	22.1	22.4	22.6	22.9	23.1	23.4	23.6
56–58	22.7	23.0	23.2	23.4	23.7	23.9	24.2	24.4	24.7
59–61	23.7	24.0	24.2	24.5	24.7	25.0	25.2	25.5	25.7
62–64	24.7	25.0	25.2	25.5	25.7	26.0	27.7	26.4	26.7
65–67	25.7	25.9	26.2	26.4	26.7	26.9	27.2	27.4	27.7
68–70	26.6	26.9	27.1	27.4	27.6	27.9	28.1	28.4	28.6
71–73	27.5	27.8	28.0	29.3	28.5	28.8	29.0	29.3	29.5
74–76	28.4	28.7	29.0	28.3	29.5	29.7	29.9	30.2	30.4
77–79	29.3	29.5	29.8	30.0	30.3	30.5	30.8	31.0	31.3
80–82	30.1	30.4	30.6	30.9	31.1	31.4	31.6	31.9	32.1
83–85	30.9	31.2	31.4	31.7	31.9	32.2	32.4	32.7	32.9
86–88	31.7	32.0	32.2	32.5	32.7	32.9	33.2	33.4	33.7
89–91	32.5	32.7	33.0	33.2	33.5	33.7	33.9	34.2	34.4
92–94	33.2	33.4	33.7	33.9	34.2	34.4	34.7	34.9	35.2
95–97	33.9	34.1	34.4	34.6	34.9	35.1	35.4	35.6	35.9
98–100	34.6	34.8	35.1	35.3	35.5	35.8	36.0	36.3	36.5
101–103	35.3	35.4	35.7	35.9	36.2	36.4	36.7	36.9	37.2
104–106	35.8	36.1	36.3	36.6	36.8	37.1	37.3	37.5	37.8
107–109	36.4	36.7	36.9	37.1	37.4	37.6	37.9	38.1	38.4
110–112	37.0	37.2	37.5	37.7	38.0	38.2	38.5	38.7	38.9
113–115	37.5	37.8	38.0	38.2	38.5	38.7	39.0	39.2	39.5

*Percent fat calculated by the Siri Formula: (% fat = $[4.95 \div BD - 4.5] \times 100$), where BD = body density

Taken from Pollock, M. L., Schmidt, D. H., and Jackson, A. S. "Measurement of Cardiorespiration Fitness and Body Composition in the Clinical Setting." *Comprehensive Therapy,* Vol. 6, September 1980.

become popular in this new era of microelectronics; many individuals have replaced vigorous activities such as cycling, hiking, and swimming with passive activities such as watching television and playing computer games. As Americans have become more sedentary, they have also become less fit and more overfat.

Another problem facing Americans is the physical education requirement in school systems. Recent studies have shown that youth are less fit today than they were a decade ago. In many schools, students experience vigorous activity only once a week, if at all. This is not sufficient to gain an adequate level of fitness. In fact, research now indicates the average adult between 30 and 40 years of age is more fit than his or her teenage counterpart. Hopefully, as Americans become better educated about the benefits of exercise with regard to fitness and weight control, this trend will be reversed.

Eating Habits.   The eating habits you develop are an important part of your weight-control program. These habits relate not only to the types of food you eat, but also to when, how, and how much you eat. Research indicates that overfat individuals tend to be more susceptible to external cues. External cues are environmental factors—other than true hunger—that may trigger you to eat. You may associate eating with watching television, reading, or listening to music. Significant emotional changes, such as anxiety or depression, may also contribute to overeating as a method to abate psychological distress. Other behavioral factors that may lead to significant weight gain are eating late at night before bedtime, high-calorie snacking, and eating rapidly. Besides increasing your caloric intake, diets high in fats, refined carbohydrates, and artificial sweeteners are thought to raise your setpoint. Behavior modification, which allows you to recognize poor eating habits and change them through a relearning process, is the best way to eliminate some of these adverse eating habits. The University of North Carolina at Chapel Hill has identified some tips for eating and grocery shopping. These include

1. Make eating a "pure" experience by engaging in no other activities, besides socializing with family and friends, while eating (i.e., no reading, TV, and so on).
2. Do all of your eating in the kitchen or dining room and then only while sitting down at your personal place at the table or counter.
3. Eliminate snacks.
4. Plan and record what you eat before you eat.
5. Pause for at least two to five minutes before beginning to eat.
6. Slow your rate of eating by placing utensils on your plate after every mouthful and not picking them up again until the food has been swallowed.
7. Measure every portion you take.
8. Make normal portions appear to be larger by using a smaller plate.
9. Make second helpings difficult to obtain.
10. Identify the people who are most likely to be of help to you. Inform them about your specific plans. Enlist their positive support.
11. Drink a glass of water ten minutes before each meal.
12. Eat whole fruit rather than drinking juice. It takes longer and is more satisfying.
13. Eat three small meals a day rather than two large meals.
14. Practice stocking only healthy low-calorie snacks in your refrigerator.
15. Prepare a list of needed items before you enter the store and buy nothing that is not on your list.

16. Shop after you have eaten a full meal.
17. Avoid browsing. Walk only through the aisles that stock the foods you need.
18. Avoid buying foods high in fat and in refined sugars. Instead, purchase foods low in fat and high in complex carbohydrates.
19. If you feel that you must buy problem foods, buy them in a form that requires the greatest possible level of preparation in the smallest possible portions.
20. Store all foods in covered containers that are kept only in the kitchen.

EATING DISORDERS

The current emphasis on physical appearance in our society has increased the frequency of eating disorders. Anorexia nervosa is now and has long been considered a serious problem. In the last several years bulimia has begun to occur with increasing frequency. Both are complex emotional disorders that could affect your psychological and physical well-being.

Anorexia nervosa is a condition characterized by deliberate self starvation with profound psychiatric and physical side effects. Common warning signs include (1) an intense fear of becoming obese that does not diminish with increased weight loss and is sometimes accompanied by a distorted body image; (2) prolonged exercise in spite of fatigue, weakness, and hyperactivity; (3) at least a 25 percent loss of original body weight without some other factor accounting for the weight loss; (4) insisting on keeping one's body weight below the minimal level for age and height norms regardless of existing percent body fat; and (5) unusual eating rituals or patterns.

Bulimia is characterized by food obsession with compulsive binge eating and purging. Binge eating is a rapid consumption of food in a short period of time. In a two-hour period as many as 5,500 calories may be consumed, with the average consumption being approximately 4,800 calories. Often the binge consists of high-calorie, easily ingested, sweet food. In addition, the individual is normally secretive about the disorder. Abdominal pain, sleep, social interruption, or self-induced vomiting usually ends the binge. Along with self-induced vomiting, the bulimic individual sometimes resorts to severely restrictive diets, laxatives, and diuretics as a means of losing weight. Because of the frequent alternation of binging, purging, and fasting, the bulimic individual experiences frequent weight fluctuations of as much as ten pounds. The individual is aware that the eating pattern is abnormal but is unable to stop eating. Often low self-esteem, stress, and depression accompany the eating binges. It is interesting to note that the bulimic individual's body weight is often normal or slightly higher than normal.

Some individuals exhibit behavior patterns that are a combination of anorexia nervosa and bulimia. These disorders appear to be more common in women than in men. The causes of these eating disorders are not readily apparent; however, certain psychological factors do play a role. These include (1) stressful life situations with which the individual is unable to cope; (2) concessions to excessive cultural pressure that often boasts that "thin is in"; (3) family gatherings centered around food; and (4) the absence of meaningful peer relationships.

A positive approach for the treatment of anorexia nervosa or bulimia is a combination of medical treatment and psychotherapy for the patient and counseling for family members. Early detection and treatment are imperative for controlling these disorders. Unfortunately, some anorexic and bulimic individuals die as a result of their disorders; some struggle with the condition for a lifetime, while others recover with no further difficulty. Professional help for both anorexia nervosa and bulimia is available at most student health and counseling centers.

PREVENTING OBESITY

Controlling your body fat and weight is a lifelong process of monitoring your diet, exercise, and eating habits. There are no easy ways to control your weight. Drugs, fancy gadgets, surgery, and drastic diets seem to promise the world to those who are desperate, but their results and safety are questionable. The most intelligent and effective method of maintaining your ideal weight and combating obesity is to eat a sensible diet and exercise on a regular basis.

Role of Exercise.   Exercise plays an important part in the battle against obesity. Dieters too often concentrate solely on dieting and neglect the role that increased physical activity can play in a weight-reduction program. The weight loss one experiences during a weight-control program consists of both fat weight and lean muscle mass. With dieting alone, approximately 30 percent of the total weight loss will be lean muscle mass; however, when exercise is combined with dieting, only 5 to 10 percent of the weight loss is lean muscle mass.

Much evidence supports the theory that physical inactivity is the factor most responsible for the increasing number of overfat people in modern Western societies. Several studies, comparing food intake and physical activity patterns of overfat individuals, attributed the fat-weight difference to a sedentary lifestyle instead of food consumption—the food intake was not significantly different for those who were overfat and those who were not. The forms of exercise found to be most helpful in a weight-reducing program were activities that demanded large caloric expenditures, such as slow long-distance running. If a weight training program is used, the exercises should be performed with light resistance and high repetitions. Table 7.4 lists numerous activities and the estimated caloric expenditure per minute/per pound for each. Although this chart provides useful estimates, actual caloric expenditures will vary based upon an individual's frame size, the intensity of the activity, and so on.

In addition to maintaining a higher percentage of lean muscle mass, exercise plays other important roles in your weight-control program. Training at least four times per week for a duration of 30 minutes per training session appears to lower the setpoint. This allows you to lose and then maintain a lower body weight and body-fat percentage. Also, during vigorous exercise, your metabolic rate may increase as much as 13 times the resting rate. Your body weight, duration of exercise, and intensity of exercise are important factors for caloric expenditure. A person who weighs 160 pounds and runs three miles in 16 minutes will burn only 5 to 10 percent more calories than by running the same distance in 24 minutes. You can burn just as many calories by training longer at a lower intensity.

Following exercise, your metabolic rate may be elevated as much as 30 to 50 calories per hour for the next six to eight hours.

CALCULATING YOUR DESIRED BODY WEIGHT

Table 7.1 enables you to classify your body composition based upon your percent body fat. The percentage of body fat you have is, in a sense, an individual choice, and the desired amount will vary from person to person. For health reasons, it is not advisable to be overfat or extremely lean. Individuals who are classified as fat tend to become overfat with age. It

Table 7.4   Caloric expenditure per minute per pound for selected activities.

Archery	.034	Making bed	.026
Baseball (except pitching)	.031	Mountain climbing	.067
Basketball	.047	Running (treadmill), 5.0 mph	.056
Bowling	.044	Running, sprinting	.155
Chopping wood	.050	Running, cross-country	.074
Circuit training, females	.045	Showering	.021
Circuit training, males	.053	Sitting, reading	.008
Classwork, lecture	.011	Sitting, writing	.012
Conversing	.012	Sleeping	.008
Cycling, 5.5 mph	.029	Squash	.069
Cycling, own pace	.045–.068	Sweeping floors	.024
Driving car	.020	Swimming, breaststroke	.074
Football	.054	Swimming, back crawl	.077
Gardening, digging	.062	Tennis	.046
Gardening, weeding	.035	Volleyball	.023
Golfing	.036	Walking, 1.15 mph	.037
House painting	.023	Walking up stairs	.052

Adapted from *Choices in Health and Fitness for Life* by S. Althoff, M. Svoboda, D. Girdano. Copyright © 1992 by Gorsuch Scarisbrick, Publishers, Scottsdale, AZ. Used with permission.

is important that you combine a balanced diet with a good exercise program to maintain your body fat at an acceptable level.

Your body weight is composed of lean body weight and fat weight. If you weigh 200 pounds and your percent body fat is 15 percent, then you have 30 pounds of fat. The other 170 pounds is considered to be lean body weight. If you decide to lower your percent body fat to 12 percent, how much should you weigh? To calculate your desired body weight, you must first calculate lean body weight and body-fat weight as we did at the beginning of this paragraph. In this example, if you want your body fat to be 12 percent of your body weight, then the present lean body mass (170 pounds) will need to represent 88 percent of your desired weight. Therefore, 170 pounds = 88 percent of your desired body weight.

You can then find your desired body weight by dividing 170 pounds by .88, which gives you a desired body weight of 193.18 pounds, composed of 12 percent fat and 88 percent lean body weight. To reach your desired body weight, you need to lose 6.82 pounds from your present body weight of 200 pounds.

Review of Steps

1. Measure your current body weight and percent body fat.
2. Determine your lean body weight and body-fat weight.
3. Decide on your desired percent body fat.
4. Divide your lean body weight by (100 percent minus desired percent body fat). This gives your desired body weight.
5. Subtract your desired body weight from your current body weight to determine how many pounds you need to lose.

GUIDELINES FOR PROPER WEIGHT REDUCTION

It is estimated that 60 to 70 million American adults and at least 10 million American teenagers are obese. Since millions of Americans have adopted unsupervised weight-loss programs, the American College of Sports Medicine feels that guidelines are needed and has issued the following outline for a weight-reduction program.

1. Prolonged fasting and diet programs that severely restrict caloric intake are scientifically undesirable and can be medically dangerous due to the loss of large amounts of water, electrolytes, minerals, glycogen stores, and other fat-free tissue (including proteins within fat-free tissue).

2. Mild caloric restriction (500 to 1,000 calories less than the usual daily intake) results in a smaller loss of water, electrolytes, minerals, and other fat-free tissue, and is less likely to cause malnutrition.

3. Dynamic exercise of large muscles (such as running, swimming, cycling, handball, and racquetball) helps to maintain fat-free tissue, including muscle mass and bone density, and results in loss of body weight. Weight loss resulting from an increase in energy expenditure is primarily in the form of fat weight.

4. A nutritionally sound diet achieving mild caloric restriction, combined with an endurance exercise program, is recommended for weight reduction. The rate of sustained weight loss should not exceed two pounds per week.

5. Maintaining proper weight control and optimal body-fat levels requires a lifetime commitment to proper eating habits and regular physical activity.

COMMONLY ASKED QUESTIONS ABOUT WEIGHT CONTROL

The following questions are commonly asked by individuals attempting to control body weight and body fat.

1. *Is it possible to spot reduce?*

   Spot reducing is possible only through surgery. When weight loss occurs in the body, fat is lost from all areas where fat is stored. However, the areas of the body with the greater amount of fat will have the greater percentage of fat loss.

2. *Is crash dieting dangerous?*

   Yes! Crash dieting implies a radical reduction in food consumption, bordering on semi-starvation. A major problem with this type of weight loss is that essential proteins, vitamins, and minerals are eliminated from the diet. Also, a large part of the weight loss from crash diets consists of protein and water from lean muscle tissue, which is replaced rapidly when eating is resumed. Most physicians agree that excess fat should be removed from the body the same way it was deposited—slowly and gradually. A reduction of two pounds per week is considered both safe and practical.

3. *Does muscle turn to fat when one stops exercising?*

   No, muscle does not turn to fat when one stops exercising or at any other time. However, belief in this myth is easy to understand when one observes a once lean and muscular individual who has become fat and flabby. What appears to be muscle changing to fat is simply the cumulative effects of long-term deconditioning and a positive caloric imbalance. The muscle cells atrophy due to inactivity, while the fat cells increase in size due to the caloric intake being greater than the caloric expenditure.

4. Does exercise increase one's appetite?

Some overfat people are apprehensive about using exercise to help reduce body fat because they are afraid exercise will increase their appetite and thus cause them to gain more body fat. However, this is not the case. Human beings were intended to be active beings. Initially, vigorous activity suppresses the appetite. After a period of time, appetite may increase, but it is not proportional to the increased caloric expenditure resulting from the increased activity.

5. Is it true that the amount of energy required to burn one pound of fat is equal to walking 35 miles or chopping wood for seven hours?

Yes, this is true. However, it is important to put these assertions into proper perspective. Walking a mile a day for 35 days or chopping wood for 15 minutes per day for a month will also take off one pound of body fat. Also, remember the caloric expenditure during recovery is not being considered in the above example.

In summary, you should consider many factors when attempting to control your body weight and percent body fat. Good eating habits, proper diet, and a vigorous exercise program all go hand in hand in this effort.

SUPPLEMENTARY READINGS

Blumenthal, J., S. Rose, and J. Chang. "Anorexia Nervosa and Exercise." *Sports Medicine,* No. 2, 1985.

D'Augelli, A. R., and W. H. Smiciklas. "The Case for Primary Prevention of Overweight Through the Family." *Journal of Nutrition Education,* April–June 1978.

Epstein, L. H., and R. R. Wing. "Aerobic Exercise and Weight," *Addictive Behaviors,* Vol. 5, 1980.

Guyton, A. C. *Textbook of Medical Physiology.* 8th ed. Philadelphia: W. B. Saunders, 1990.

Hager, A. "Nutritional Problems in Adolescence—Obesity." *Nutrition Reviews,* February 1981.

Hanna, C. H., et al. "Differences in the Degree of Overweight: A Note of Its Importance." *Addictive Behaviors,* 1981.

Hargetetal, B. S. "The Caloric Cost of Running." *Journal of the American Medical Association,* Vol. 8, 1974.

Hertzler, A. A. "Obesity—Impact on Family." *Journal of the American Dietetic Association,* November 1981.

Keys, A. "Overweight, Obesity, Coronary Heart Disease and Mortality." *Nutrition Reviews,* September 1980.

Marley, W. P. *Health and Physical Fitness.* Dubuque, IA: Wm. C. Brown, 1988.

Metropolitan Life Insurance Company. "New Weight Standards for Men and Women." *Statistical Bulletin,* 1983.

Neuman, P., and P. Halvorson. *Anorexia Nervosa and Bulimia: A Handbook for Counselors and Therapists.* New York: Van Nostrand Reinhold, 1983.

Rodin, J., and J. Slochower. "Externality in the Nonobese: Effects of Environmental Responsiveness on Weight." *Journal of Personality and Social Psychology,* Vol. 33, 1976.

Shils, M. E., et al., eds. *Modern Nutrition in Health & Disease.* 8th ed. Baltimore, MD: Williams & Wilkins, 1993.

University of North Carolina Health Services. *Aids for Eating More Sensibly.* February 1981.

CHAPTER 7 REVIEW QUESTIONS

1. Obesity is being _____ , not _____ .

2. List two major hazards of obesity.
   a.

   b.

3. When does obesity occur?

4. What is creeping obesity?

5. Lowering the setpoint can be accomplished by
   a.

   b.

   c.

   d.

6. What are the two types of fat cells in the body?

7. List five things you can do to help yourself not overeat.

   a.

   b.

   c.

   d.

   e.

8. What is anorexia nervosa?

9. What is bulimia?

10. What would be a positive approach for the treatment of anorexia nervosa or bulimia?

11. Controlling your body fat is a lifelong process of monitoring your

    a.

    b.

    c.

12. What role does exercise play in the battle against obesity?

13. _____ is the factor most responsible for the increasing number of overfat people in modern Western societies.

14. Training at least _____ times per week for a duration of _____ minutes per training session appears to lower the setpoint.

15. During vigorous exercise, your metabolic rate may increase as much as _____ times the resting rate.

16. List five guidelines for proper weight reduction.

    a.

    b.

    c.

    d.

    e.

17. Larry Lazy weighs 220 pounds and has 20 percent body fat. If he would like to have 13 percent body fat, what would be his desired body weight?

CHAPTER

8

Stress Management

During the course of any day, you make a number of decisions while balancing demands of school, work, personal and family relationships, and even leisure activities. Although these demands are part of everyday life, they may add stress to your life. This chapter will help you deal with stress more effectively.

WHAT IS STRESS?

The term *stress* has many definitions. Some researchers define stress as anything that threatens the existence of an organism. Others describe stress as an upset of the homeostatic balance of the body caused by psychic, physical, or social conditions. A moderate level of stress is desirable—it prepares the body to react to the stress-causing event and improves performance. However, too much stress will result in a decrease in performance and health. Stress can have a positive or negative effect, depending upon your ability to cope.

PHYSICAL RESPONSES TO STRESS

How does the body respond to stressful situations? The bodily responses to stress vary among individuals. Different emotional states activate the release of epinephrine and norepinephrine from the adrenal medulla. These hormones can increase the body's capacity to perform vigorous muscular activity by (1) increasing arterial pressure; (2) increasing blood flow to the active muscles and decreasing the blood flow to organs not needed for rapid activity; (3) increasing the rates of cellular metabolism throughout the body; (4) increasing the blood glucose concentration; (5) increasing glycolysis in the muscle; (6) increasing muscular strength; (7) increasing mental activity; and (8) increasing the rate of blood coagulation. These are positive adaptive responses triggered by different stimuli. However, if these responses are not immediately followed by vigorous exercise, a number of negative things can happen to the body. These include (1) constant low-level strain on the cardiovascular system that can lead to heart disease; (2) an increased cholesterol level combined with a decreased ability to clear the blood of this cholesterol; and (3) an increased tendency for the clotting elements of the blood to fall out and settle onto the walls of the veins and arteries.

Vigorous muscular activity will enhance the conversion of fatty acids into energy before they collect along the arterial walls. However, lack of vigorous muscular activity increases the chance of atherosclerotic development.

Physical cues often signal the onset of stress; these cues vary from one person to another and include tightening of neck muscles, minor headaches, or an upset stomach. Other physical responses include loss of appetite, inability to sleep, and a disruption of bodily functions. In addition, if continually aroused by stress, you are more likely to develop high blood pressure, ulcers, diabetes, and colitis.

BEHAVIORAL PATTERNS

The behavioral patterns you develop may have a positive or negative influence on the way that you handle stress. Generally, behavioral patterns are broken into three classes, which we'll call Types A, B, and C.

Type A individuals are typically overachievers, excessively competitive, constantly impatient, hard-driving, high-strung, and harboring free-floating hostility. On the other hand, Type B individuals are usually relaxed and easygoing. The traits of the Type B individual are almost exactly opposite those of the Type A individual. Type C individuals possess the same traits as Type A except they do not harbor feelings of hostility.

Until recently, there was no distinction between Type A and Type C behavior. Epidemiologists realized that people who were Type A had a much higher incidence of coronary heart disease than did Type B people. However, these were the Type A individuals with feelings of anger and hostility. Those without feelings of anger and hostility had incidence rates of coronary heart disease comparable to their Type B counterparts. These individuals have been reclassified as Type C. These individuals normally are hard-driving, highly competitive overachievers, and often participate in a regular fitness program to keep themselves physically prepared for the demands placed upon them.

MANAGING STRESS

Understanding your behavior patterns and realizing that stress can exact a severe toll on your health are important factors in behavior modification. Behavioral patterns, including those classified as Type A, are learned and developed.

To bring about a change in your ability to handle stress, you may need to *alter your perspective on life*. How you perceive life's situations determines whether an event is stressful to you or not. Often two individuals will view the same event in different ways; one individual may experience a high level of stress, while the other may experience very little stress. The example of two students preparing for an English exam demonstrates this point. One approaches the exam as a necessary step in his preparation to become an engineer. The second student is upset about the exam—she perceives it as a waste of time because her goal is to become an engineer, not an English major. Both face the same task, but view it differently.

You cannot assume that others are responsible for your problems. Failure to take responsibility for your own problems will not solve them. There is merit in the old saying "Look in a mirror and you can usually find both the cause and solution for your problems." To a great degree, we are what we want to be.

In your dealings with other people, *try to be understanding and attempt to see the other person's point of view.* Realize that most people have good reasons for their positions.

Develop the ability to look at the big picture. Incidents often seem extremely important to us at the time they occur. However, attempt to analyze them within a larger time frame and they will usually appear less important and not so traumatic. An example of this may be an individual who fails at a given task. No one enjoys performing poorly. However, it will be less important as time passes. It is important to realize that you, like everyone else, are going to experience a few disappointments during your life. You need to develop an appreciation for the simple things so that you will be able to handle the disappointments that you may experience. Take time each day to reflect upon life's gifts and beauty. Life is generally what we make of it.

Mental and muscle relaxation methods eliminate stress. You can attain mental relaxation by finding a quiet place where you can sit or lie comfortably and close your eyes. Once in this position, listening to soothing music may help. Combining mental relaxation techniques with muscular relaxation often helps. The muscular relaxation method consists of attempting to tense a muscle group and then relaxing it. Start with your toes and work toward your head. Try to focus your attention on the soothing feeling of relaxation that follows the muscle tension. Relax each muscle group of the body this way. You can also use slow deep breathing and sighing techniques for relaxation. Other methods for relaxation include meditation and self-suggestion techniques.

Physical exercise may play a major role in helping to combat stress. The mind and the body are intimately linked with your health. Exercise is very important to the human body in managing stress. Vigorous exercise helps relieve muscular tension and helps return epinephrine and norepinephrine levels to normal. Many students use the early evening hours as their time for exercise in order to relieve the stress that mounts during the day. By dissipating the stress that you accumulated during the day, you are better able to handle your studies at night.

You can often convert anger or tension to muscle relaxation experienced after sustained physical exertion. Vigorous exercise may also lessen the feeling of anxiety that may be present before an important event. The physical benefits derived from exercise are just as important as the mental ones. Good muscle tone and an improved cardiovascular system reduce the physiological problems that can develop as a result of stressful situations.

MEASURING STRESS AND TENSION

These three tests were developed by the Public Health Service of the former U.S. Department of Health, Education, and Welfare (now the Department of Health and Human Services). The first two parts are designed to give you an indication of how vulnerable you might be to certain types of stress and to make you aware of how they might affect you. The last part of the test will provide you with information on how to cope with situations that might be of a stressful nature. Additional information regarding these tests can be found in Department of Health and Human Services Publication No. (PHS) 79-50097, Washington, D.C., 1980.

Test One

Choose the most appropriate answer for each of the ten questions as it actually pertains to you.

1. *When I can't do something "my way," I simply adjust and do it the easiest way.*

    (a) Almost always true (b) Usually true (c) Usually false (d) Almost always false

2. **I get upset when someone in front of me drives slowly.**
    (a) Almost always true (b) Usually true (c) Usually false (d) Almost always false

3. **It bothers me when my plans are dependent upon others.**
    (a) Almost always true (b) Usually true (c) Usually false (d) Almost always false

4. **Whenever possible, I tend to avoid large crowds.**
    (a) Almost always true (b) Usually true (c) Usually false (d) Almost always false

5. **I am uncomfortable when I have to stand in long lines.**
    (a) Almost always true (b) Usually true (c) Usually false (d) Almost always false

6. **Arguments upset me.**
    (a) Almost always true (b) Usually true (c) Usually false (d) Almost always false

7. **When my plans don't flow smoothly, I become anxious.**
    (a) Almost always true (b) Usually true (c) Usually false (d) Almost always false

8. **I require a lot of space in which to live and work.**
    (a) Almost always true (b) Usually true (c) Usually false (d) Almost always false

9. **When I am busy at some task, I hate to be disturbed.**
    (a) Almost always true (b) Usually true (c) Usually false (d) Almost always false

10 **I believe that it is worth waiting for all good things.**
    (a) Almost always true (b) Usually true (c) Usually false (d) Almost always false

To score: 1 and 10, a = 1 pt., b = 2 pts., c = 3 pts., d = 4 pts.; 2 through 9, a = 4 pts., b = 3 pts., c = 2 pts., d = 1 pt.

Test One measures your vulnerability to stress from being frustrated or inhibited. Scores in excess of 25 seem to suggest some vulnerability to this source of stress.

Test Two

Answer each question as it is generally true for you.

1. **I hate to wait in lines.**
    (a) Almost always true (b) Usually true (c) Seldom true (d) Never true

2. **I often find myself racing against the clock to save time.**
    (a) Almost always true (b) Usually true (c) Seldom true (d) Never true

3. **I become upset if I think something is taking too long.**
    (a) Almost always true (b) Usually true (c) Seldom true (d) Never true

4. **When under pressure, I tend to lose my temper.**
    (a) Almost always true (b) Usually true (c) Seldom true (d) Never true

5. **My friends tell me that I tend to get irritated easily.**
    (a) Almost always true (b) Usually true (c) Seldom true (d) Never true

6. **I seldom like to do anything unless I can make it competitive.**
    (a) Almost always true (b) Usually true (c) Seldom true (d) Never true

7. **When something must be done, I'm the first to begin even though the details may still need to be worked out.**
   (a) Almost always true (b) Usually true (c) Seldom true (d) Never true

8. **When I make a mistake, it is usually because I've rushed into something without giving it enough thought and planning.**
   (a) Almost always true (b) Usually true (c) Seldom true (d) Never true

9. **Whenever possible, I try to do two things at once, such as eating while working, or planning while driving or bathing.**
   (a) Almost always true (b) Usually true (c) Seldom true (d) Never true

10. **When I go on a vacation, I usually take along some work to do just in case I get a chance.**
    (a) Almost always true (b) Usually true (c) Seldom true (d) Never true

To score: a = 4 pts., b = 3 pts., c = 2 pts., d = 1 pt.

This test measures the presence of compulsive, time-urgent, and excessively aggressive behavioral traits. Scores in excess of 25 suggest the presence of one or more of these traits.

Test Three

This test was created largely on the basis of results compiled by clinicians and researchers who sought to identify how individuals effectively cope with stress. This test is an educational tool, not a clinical instrument. Its purpose, therefore, is to inform you of ways in which you can effectively and healthfully cope with the stress in your life. At the same time, through a point system, it will give you some indication of the relative desirability of the coping strategies you are currently using. Simply follow the instructions given for each of the 14 items listed. Total your points when you have completed all of the items.

1. Give yourself 10 points if you feel that you have a supportive family.
2. Give yourself 10 points if you actively pursue a hobby.
3. Give yourself 10 points if you belong to some social or activity group that meets at least once a month (other than your family).
4. Give yourself 15 points if you are within five pounds of your ideal body weight, considering your height and bone structure.
5. Give yourself 15 points if you practice some form of deep relaxation at least three times a week. Deep-relaxation exercises include meditation, imagery, yoga, and similar activities.
6. Give yourself 5 points for each time you exercise 30 minutes or longer during an average week.
7. Give yourself 5 points for each nutritionally balanced and wholesome meal you consume during an average day.
8. Give yourself 5 points if you do something just for yourself that you really enjoy during an average week.
9. Give yourself 10 points if you have some place in your home that you can go in order to relax and/or be alone.
10. Give yourself 10 points if you practice time management techniques in your daily life.

11. Subtract 10 points for each pack of cigarettes you smoke during one average day.

12. Subtract 5 points for each evening during an average week that you take any form of medication or chemical substance (including alcohol) to help you sleep.

13. Subtract 10 points for each day during an average week that you consume any form of medication or chemical substance (including alcohol) to reduce your anxiety or just to calm you down.

14. Subtract 5 points for each evening during an average week that you bring work home—work that was meant to be done at your place of employment.

Now calculate your total score. A "perfect" score would be 115 points or more. If you scored in the 50-to-60 range you probably have an adequate collection of coping strategies for most common sources of stress. You should keep in mind, however, that the higher your score, the greater your ability to cope with stress.

SUPPLEMENTARY READINGS

Blumenthal, J. "Relaxation Therapy, Biofeedback, and Behavioral Medicine." *Psychotherapy,* Vol. 22, No. 3, 1985.

Blumenthal, J., S. Rose, and J. Chang. "Anorexia Nervosa and Exercise." *Sports Medicine,* No. 2, 1985.

Charlesworth, E., and R. Nathan. "How to Build a Healthy Response to Stress." *Advertising Age,* Vol. 56, 1985.

Cottrell, R. *Wellness: Stress Management.* Guilford, CT: Dushkin Publishing Group, 1992.

Duke Health Line, Vol. 1, 1985.

Gil, K., and J. Blumenthal. "Behavior Modification in the Primary and Secondary Prevention of Coronary Heart Disease." *Cardiology in Practice,* Vol. 1, No. 6, 1985.

Greenberg, J. *Your Personal Stress Profile.* Dubuque, IA: William C. Brown Publishers. 1992.

Guyton, A. C. *Textbook of Medical Physiology.* 8th ed. Philadelphia: W. B. Saunders, 1990.

Kleiner, B., and S. Geil. "Managing Stress Effectively." *Journal of Systems Management,* 1985.

Kriegel, R. J., and M. H. Kriegel. *The C Zone: Peak Performance Under Pressure.* New York: Fawcett, 1985.

Nieman, D. C. *Fitness and Your Health.* Palo Alto, CA: Bull Publishing Company, 1993.

Pascarella, P. "Job Stress: A State of Mind." *Industry Week,* Nov. 29, 1982.

Seaward, B. L. *Managing Stress: Principles and Strategies for Health and Well-being.* Boston: Jones and Bartlett Publishers, 1994.

Seiger, L. H., and J. Hesson. *Walking For Fitness.* 2d ed. Madison, WI: Brown & Benchmark, 1994.

CHAPTER 8 REVIEW QUESTIONS

1. What is stress?

2. Is stress good or bad?

3. The release of epinephrine and norepinephrine from the adrenal medulla can increase the body's capacity to perform vigorous muscular activity by
   a.

   b.

   c.

   d.

   e.

   f.

   g.

   h.

4. If the responses listed above are not immediately followed by vigorous exercise, a number of negative things can happen to the body, including

   a.

   b.

   c.

5. List and describe the three classes of behavioral patterns.

   a.

   b.

   c.

6. List three things you can do to help manage stress.

   a.

   b.

   c.

Appendix A:
Exercise-Related Injuries

Exercise on a regular basis is associated with improvement in many aspects of both physical and mental health. Occasionally, however, exercise may result in adverse physical changes. This is particularly the case if the exercise has resulted in an injury of the musculoskeletal system. The musculoskeletal system consists of the bones, joints, ligaments, muscles, tendons, and nerves. A properly working musculoskeletal system allows us to perform our occupational tasks and the movements that are required in sport activities. When the musculoskeletal system is stressed repeatedly during exercise, it is usually capable of adapting to the stress. The adaption to the repeated stress of exercise generally results in a strengthening of the structures involved. The most obvious example is the muscle. Regular bouts of exercise will clearly result in increased strength and endurance of the muscles being exercised. Although less noticeable, a similar process occurs in virtually every component of the musculoskeletal system in response to exercise. Bones will acquire more mass and become more dense in response to exercise. Ligaments and tendons usually become mechanically stronger as compared with nonexercised tendons and ligaments.

At times, the stress that exercise places upon the musculoskeletal system can exceed the system's capability to adapt to this stress. This will lead to a breakdown of the system that manifests itself as an injury. This appendix will discuss the most common forms of exercise-related injuries of the musculoskeletal system.

ACUTE INJURIES

In acute injuries the stress clearly exceeds the strength of the system. This causes an injury to a structure that was previously entirely normal. Acute injuries are usually associated with obvious mishaps during the exercise. The majority of the injuries are caused by accidental falls, sudden failures of exercise equipment, collisions with others, and improper use of protective equipment. The pain and disability are usually immediate, and medical attention is generally needed the day of injury. The initial approach to acute injuries is characterized by the principle of **Double RICE.** Double RICE stands for **R**est, **I**ce, **C**ompression, and **E**levation followed by **R**ehabilitate your **I**njury, then **C**ontinue your **E**xercise program. Rest is accomplished by stopping the exercise and immobilizing the injured extremity to prevent further injury. Application of ice or other cooling devices will slow down the metabolism in the injured area, which limits the damage to the tissues. In addition, it slows transmission by the nerves, which results in pain relief. Icing is usually performed by applying a plastic bag filled with ice directly to the injured area for 10 to 20 minutes. Care must be taken to avoid frostbite by placing a towel between the ice and the exposed skin. Compression will help decrease the swelling. The most common form of compression is an elastic or Ace® bandage. Elevation will work in conjunction with compression to avoid some of the swelling. Placing the injured limb above the level of the heart improves the drainage of blood and fluid from the limb. After this initial management, the injury needs to be evaluated by qualified medical personnel to determine diagnosis and treatment. You should always rehabilitate your injury before trying to continue your exercise program. Sprains, strains, and fractures are the most common acute injuries.

Sprains.   Sprains are acute partial or complete tears of the ligaments. Ligaments are strong fibrous bands that connect bone to bone and provide stability in our joints. Some joints, such as the knee, obtain the majority of their stability from ligaments. Others, such as the hip joint, are quite stable already because of the ball and socket configuration of the joint and the strong muscles that surround the joint. The most common sprains occur in the knee and ankle. In the knee, complete ligament tears can lead to chronic instability because the knee is dependent on the ligaments for stability. Knee ligament surgery may be needed in some injuries to correct this problem.

Ankle sprains or ankle ligament tears usually result from a twisting injury to the joint, such as stepping on an uneven surface. Most ankle sprains are partial ligament tears. The micro-tears of the ligament in the ankle will normally heal quite well with appropriate immobilization of the joint, and surgery is rarely needed. Usually, it will take four to six weeks before the pain and swelling have disappeared.

Strains.   Strains are acute partial or complete tears of the muscle–tendon unit. Muscles are capable of contracting, thereby bringing about movement of our extremities. Their contractile power is transferred through the tendons to the bones. Tendons appear very similar to ligaments but connect muscles to bones instead of connecting two bones. A sudden acute stretch of the muscle–tendon unit during activity can result in a strain injury, especially if the muscle was contracting at the same time. Muscles that are particularly susceptible to strains are the back of the upper leg, or hamstring group, and back of the lower leg, or calf muscles. Fortunately, most strains are partial instead of complete tears. However, if the tears are complete, as sometimes occur in the rotator cuff of the shoulder or the Achilles tendon at the back of the heel, surgery may be needed to repair the injury. Most significant strains take at least six weeks to heal.

Fractures.   Fractures are complete or incomplete breaks of the bone. Most fractures are caused by a direct impact at the site of injury. Fortunately, the force needed to fracture a healthy bone is often quite large. Sprains and strains are therefore much more common in sport participants than fractures. Fractures cause immediate pain, swelling, and inability to use the involved extremity. Because of the risks of further displacing the fractured bone ends, individuals suffering fractures should normally be transported by qualified personnel to an appropriate facility for evaluation and treatment. Bone healing normally requires from four to ten weeks.

CHRONIC INJURIES

In chronic injuries, the damage to the involved structure does not occur in a single episode as it does in acute injuries. Chronic injuries develop during repeated exercise sessions in which the stress each time is just enough to exceed the limits of the structure. This causes a small or micro-injury to the musculoskeletal structure. If several strenuous exercise sessions take place within a short time span, the micro-injuries in the structure do not have time to heal, and the structure cannot gradually adapt by becoming stronger. The small but excessive and repeated stress produces small injuries that slowly but surely accumulate into a more severe injury.

Often an error in training or use of equipment is associated with these injuries. A sudden change or increase in workout routines can be the culprit, since the body does not have enough time to adapt to the change. Worn or inappropriate shoes are a common equipment problem that may cause chronic overuse injuries such as shin splints, pain radiating from the heel of the foot, or pain radiating from the arch at the bottom of the foot. Unfortunately, by the time the pain of the injury manifests itself, the process has usually been ongoing for a lengthy period of time.

The general principles of treatment for these injuries involve a decrease of the exercise intensity and/or frequency (relative rest) and a review of the equipment being used. The relative rest allows the structure to do some "catch-up healing" and slowly adapt to the exercise by becoming stronger. Absolute rest is often not needed or even not advisable since it takes away the stimulus for the structure to slowly adapt and become stronger. New, well-cushioned shoes can solve footwear problems. Many individuals use ice application after workout sessions and anti-inflammatory medication such as ibuprofen and aspirin to decrease the presumed inflammatory response associated with these injuries. Care should be taken to ensure that you do not overuse the anti-inflammatory medication. Stretching helps keep the structure flexible and thereby less susceptible to repeated injury. Once the initial pain and inflammation have subsided, the intensity and frequency can be increased again. This should be done gradually since flare-ups are frequent while recovering from an overuse injury.

Common chronic injuries include muscle soreness, blisters, tendinitis, shin splints, and stress fractures. These injuries can be avoided by gradually increasing the stress encountered in your exercise sessions. Ensure that your training progression is not too fast. Let your body have the time it needs for rest between sessions and alternate hard and easy workout days.

Muscle Soreness.   Although muscle soreness is related to repeated exercise, it may not represent a true injury. If an untrained muscle is subjected to a strenuous exercise session, it often develops soreness that is most pronounced at approximately 48 hours following the exercise session. Research indicates that there is some damage within the muscle but this may only involve muscle cells that were already in need of replacement by the body. The muscle soreness recovers without assistance and does not recur once the muscle has become accustomed to the exercise. There are no known ways to prevent muscle soreness other than being careful to gradually increase exercise intensity.

Blisters.   Blisters are among the most common forms of injury to the skin. They are caused by excessive and repeated friction against the skin. Blisters usually occur inside shoes or tight pieces of clothing. If the friction occurs gradually, the skin will adapt and often form a callus. A callus is an area of thickened skin that is effective in withstanding friction. If the skin's rate of adaptation is exceeded, however, the superficial skin layers will separate and fluid will collect between the layers. The most superficial layer will eventually fall off and a new layer formed underneath. It is usually of little benefit to puncture the blister, since this can increase the chance of infection before the new layer has formed and has not been shown to increase the rate of healing. You should take notice of areas of increased friction and then eliminate the friction as much as possible. Proper shoe size, proper clothing, and application of a lubricant such as petroleum jelly (Vaseline®) can help prevent blisters.

Tendinitis.   Repeated microtrauma to the tendon and the surrounding tissues is generally called tendinitis. Excessive stress on the tendon can cause small injuries inside the tendon and inflammation in the sheath around the tendon. Occasionally some swelling is visible due to this inflammation, but the most common symptom is pain directly in the area of the tendon. The pain is usually present when the exercise is started but then often seems to improve somewhat. The pain again worsens after the exercise session and is usually bad the next morning because the inflammation has had time to develop. In chronic and unrecognized cases, the injury can occasionally progress to a complete rupture of the tendon. Tendons commonly susceptible to tendinitis are the Achilles tendon, the tendon between the kneecap and tibia (patellar tendinitis or jumper's knee), and the tendons of the rotator cuff muscles in the shoulder. As mentioned before, treatment is aimed at decreasing the stress in the tendon during exercise by relative rest and careful stretching. Recovery can often require several weeks before exercise intensity can gradually be increased again.

CARDIORESPIRATORY PROGRESS CHART

Name _____ Date _____

DATE	TYPE OF EXERCISE	PREEXERCISE HEART RATE	EXERCISE TIME	TARGET HEART RATE	EXERCISE DISTANCE	POSTEXERCISE HEART RATE

Appendix B:
Fitness Forms

PREEXERCISE MEDICAL AND FITNESS INFORMATION

_____   _____   _____   _____
NAME (Last)   (First)   SEX   AGE   STUDENT ID NO.

_____   _____   _____   _____   _____
COURSE   HOUR/DAY   SEMESTER/YR   LOCAL PHONE #   HOMETOWN/STATE

Introduction: Participation in a regular aerobics or strength training program has proven to provide many health benefits. However, due to the small but real health risk of participation in any fitness testing or exercise program, it is necessary to determine any contraindicators prior to this course. If any of these conditions apply, you should report them to your instructor, who may have you consult the student health services staff. Also, if you experience any medical difficulties during the semester, report them to your instructor as soon as possible.

1. How many days per week do you exercise? _____

2. How many minutes per session do you normally exercise? _____

3. How intense (mild, moderate, or vigorous) is your workout? _____

4. List the activities that your fitness program presently includes:

   a. _____   b. _____

   c. _____   d. _____

   e. _____   f. _____

   g. _____   h. _____

5. Why do you exercise? _____

6. In which areas would you like to improve the most? Please rank each area, placing a *1* by the most important area, a *2* by the next most important, and so on.

   _____ cardiorespiratory fitness   _____ percent body fat

   _____ muscular strength/endurance   _____ body image

   _____ flexibility   _____ other: _____

7. Do you smoke cigarettes? _____

8. List all medications that you are presently taking:

   a. _____   b. _____   c. _____

   d. _____   e. _____   f. _____

9. Indicate any serious injuries or hospital care in your medical history, and give approximate dates:

_____

_____

_____

10. From your understanding of this course, your physical activity background, and your medical history, do you foresee any potential problems that may limit your activity in this course?

    No _____ Yes _____ If yes, please explain. _____

11. Indicate any conditions that you have experienced in your past or present medical history:

PAST	PRESENT	CONDITION	EXPLANATION
_____	_____	Heart problems	_____
_____	_____	High blood pressure	_____
_____	_____	High blood-cholesterol levels	_____
_____	_____	Low blood sugar	_____
_____	_____	Diabetes	_____
_____	_____	Respiratory problems	_____
_____	_____	Asthma	_____
_____	_____	Joint, bone, or muscle problems	_____
_____	_____	Arthritis	_____
_____	_____	Low back pain	_____
_____	_____	Anorexia or bulimia	_____
_____	_____	Severe or frequent headaches	_____
_____	_____	Dizziness or fainting	_____
_____	_____	Stroke	_____
_____	_____	Epilepsy	_____
_____	_____	Emotional or mental problems	_____
_____	_____	Mononucleosis	_____
_____	_____	Recent operation or illness	_____
_____	_____	Other:	_____

12. What was the date of your last medical exam? _____

I, _____ hereby certify that the above is
              (Print Name)
correct to the best of my knowledge.

_____   _____
          (Date)   (Signature)

FITNESS EVALUATION RECORD

Date _____   Week # _____

Name _____   Age _____   Gender _____

Flexibility

Sit-and-Reach _____ inches

Cardiorespiratory

Resting Heart Rate_____

Step Test: EoT_____   +1 _____   +2 _____

1.5-mile run: Time _____ : _____ EoT _____+1 _____+2 _____

3.0-mile run: Time _____ : _____ EoT _____+1 _____+2 _____

Muscular Strength/Endurance

Bench Press: Resistance _____ Number of Repetitions _____

Estimated Max for Bench Press _____
(formula on page 3)

Lat Pulls: Resistance _____ Number of Repetitions _____

Estimated Max for Lat Pulls _____
(formula on page 3)

Leg Press: Resistance _____ Number of Repetitions _____

Estimated Max for Leg Press _____
(formula on page 3)

Pull-ups _____   Sit-ups _____   Crunches _____

Body Composition

Skinfolds: Thigh _____   Abd/Hip _____   Chest/Arm _____ Sum _____

Percent Fat _____(refer to Tables 7.2 and 7.3)   Body Weight _____

Desired Body Weight _____

FITNESS EVALUATION RECORD

Date _____   Week # _____

Name _____   Age _____   Gender _____

Flexibility

Sit-and-Reach _____ inches

Cardiorespiratory

Resting Heart Rate _____

Step Test: EoT _____   +1 _____   +2 _____

1.5-mile run: Time _____: _____ EoT _____ +1 _____ +2 _____

3.0-mile run: Time _____: _____ EoT _____ +1 _____ +2 _____

Muscular Strength/Endurance

Bench Press: Resistance _____ Number of Repetitions _____

Estimated Max for Bench Press _____
(formula on page 3)

Lat Pulls: Resistance _____ Number of Repetitions _____

Estimated Max for Lat Pulls   _____
(formula on page 3)

Leg Press: Resistance _____ Number of Repetitions _____

Estimated Max for Leg Press _____
(formula on page 3)

Pull-ups _____   Sit-ups _____   Crunches _____

Body Composition

Skinfolds: Thigh _____ Abd/Hip _____ Chest/Arm _____ Sum _____

Percent Fat _____ (refer to Tables 7.2 and 7.3)   Body Weight _____

Desired Body Weight _____

CARDIORESPIRATORY START SHEET

Name _____ Date _____

Target Heart Rate Zone

Lower Limit   = 60% (MHR _____ – RHR _____) + RHR _____

= 60% (_____) + _____

= _____ bpm ÷ 6 = _____ for a ten-second count

Upper Limit   = 90% (MHR _____ – RHR _____) + RHR _____

= 90% (_____) + _____

= _____ bpm ÷ 6 = _____ for a ten-second count

Exercise Intensity Check

After a complete warm-up, jog at a pace slow enough that you can still talk. After three minutes, stop and check your pulse rate for ten seconds. You should be within your target heart rate zone, but nearer the lower limit than the upper limit. Adjust your pace as indicated by your heart rate. If your heart rate is too fast, jog slower. If your heart rate is too slow, jog faster. Jog five more minutes and then repeat the heart rate check. Adjust your pace as needed. If you are just starting an exercise program, keep your heart rate near the lower limit of the target heart rate zone. If you have been working out for several weeks, you can gradually increase the intensity.

Heart rate after three minutes of jogging: _____ for a ten-second count

Indicated change in pace: Slower _____   Faster _____   No Change _____

Heart rate after five additional minutes of jogging: _____ for a ten-second count

Indicated change in pace: Slower _____   Faster _____   No Change _____

Upon completion of exercise, cool down by walking slowly and performing stretching exercises. Take your postexercise heart rate and record below.

Recovery Heart Rate: EoT _____ +1 _____ +2 _____ +3 _____ +5 _____

CARDIORESPIRATORY PROGRESS CHART

Name _____   Date _____

DATE	TYPE OF EXERCISE	PREEXERCISE HEART RATE	EXERCISE TIME	TARGET HEART RATE	EXERCISE DISTANCE	POSTEXERCISE HEART RATE

Shin Splints.   Pain in the area of the shins is a common problem if exercise intensity or frequency is increased too quickly. It is believed that a large number of athletes and exercise enthusiasts with shin splints develop an injury in the area where the muscle attaches to the bone. Most of the strong muscles that power the foot during take-off and landing are located in the lower leg. Excessive running or jumping can lead to small micro-tears in the attachment of these muscles to the tibia, resulting in a deep throbbing ache directly along the tibia during and after exercise. Be aware that stress fractures and tendinitis in this area can cause similar symptoms. Treatment includes icing the involved area after exercise, wearing well-cushioned and supportive shoes, and following a stretching program for the muscles involved. Preventive measures include gradual lower-leg warm-up. Calf-tendon stretching using the following exercise may help prevent shin splints: Stand on a stairstep and slowly rise high on your toes, then slowly lower your heels past the step edge. Repeat the stretch eight to ten times.

Stress Fractures.   Repeated stress on the bone can also slowly accumulate and result in a cracking of the bone itself. This is analogous to a fatigue crack in a piece of metal when it is bent back and forth many times. If the stress fracture is not recognized and the repeated stress is continued, the crack can be completed all the way through the bone and result in a regular acute fracture. The symptoms of a stress fracture include pain in a small area directly over the part of the bone that is involved. Unlike tendinitis, the pain is always worsened by exercise and does not improve until the involved bone is rested. Bones commonly involved in stress fractures are the metatarsal bone in the forefoot, the tibia, and the femur near the hip joint. When a stress fracture is suspected, X-rays or even a bone scan are needed to diagnose the problem. Once diagnosed, relative rest that avoids impact exercise is usually enough to allow healing of the stress fracture. Swimming and cycling are good examples of non-impact exercises and should supplement your training program to provide relative rest from chronic injuries from impact activities. However, stress fractures of the hip are often treated with surgery. The risk of completing a hip crack into an acute fracture is high due to the stress placed on the hip joint even during regular walking.

REHABILITATION

Several basic principles are followed during the rehabilitation process. The initial rehabilitation phase of a musculoskeletal injury is focused on decreasing the aftereffects of the injury. Residual pain and swelling are usually treated with mild analgesics, icing, and compression. The next step is to regain motion and flexibility through gentle but persistent stretching. When motion and flexibility are regained, you should concentrate on regaining strength and endurance through appropriate exercises. Once an acute or chronic injury has healed, it is generally not advisable to immediately resume exercise at the same level as you were at the time the injury occurred. During the healing process of an injury, not only the injured structures but also the other structures of the affected extremity decline in motion, flexibility, strength, and endurance. Rapid resumption of exercise after the injury has healed often leads to a recurrence of the original injury or other, new injuries in different parts of the body. Besides concentration on regaining the motion, flexibility, strength, and endurance in the injured parts, rehabilitation should also include uninjured parts in order to prevent these new injuries. Finally, only when the strength and endurance have started to return can actual "sports-specific" rehabilitation begin. This means a gradual, controlled return to specific activities that are required for a specific sport or activity. Following these principles can minimize new injuries or flare-up of the original injury.

MUSCULAR STRENGTH/ENDURANCE TRAINING RECORD

Name: _____   Body Weight: _____

Date: _____   Resting Heart Rate: _____

EXERCISE	SET 1 Weight × reps	SET 2 Weight × reps	SET 3 Weight × reps	SET 4 Weight × reps	SET 5 Weight × reps	TOTAL Poundange
1						
2						
3						
4						
5						
6						
7						
8						
9						
10						
11						
12						

AEROBIC EXERCISE

TYPE _____   DISTANCE _____

DURATION _____   INTENSITY _____

NUTRITIONAL INFORMATION

BREAKFAST _____

LUNCH _____

DINNER _____

COMMENTS ON WORKOUT

MUSCULAR STRENGTH/ENDURANCE TRAINING RECORD

Name: _____   Body Weight: _____

Date: _____   Resting Heart Rate: _____

EXERCISE	SET 1 Weight × reps	SET 2 Weight × reps	SET 3 Weight × reps	SET 4 Weight × reps	SET 5 Weight × reps	TOTAL Poundange
1						
2						
3						
4						
5						
6						
7						
8						
9						
10						
11						
12						

AEROBIC EXERCISE

    TYPE   _____   DISTANCE   _____

    DURATION   _____   INTENSITY   _____

NUTRITIONAL INFORMATION

    BREAKFAST   _____

    LUNCH   _____

    DINNER   _____

COMMENTS ON WORKOUT

Index